Shrink Yourself

Shrink Yourself

Break Free from Emotional Eating Forever

ROGER GOULD, M.D.

WILEY

John Wiley & Sons, Inc.

Published by John Wiley & Sons, Inc., Hoboken, New Jersey
Published simultaneously in Canada

Design and composition by Navta Associates, Inc.

The information contained in this book is not intended to serve as a replacement for professional medical advice. Any use of the information in this book is at the reader's discretion. The author and the publisher specifically disclaim any and all liability arising directly or indirectly from the use or application of any information contained in this book. A health care professional should be consulted regarding your specific situation.

For general information about our other products and services, please contact our Customer Care Department within the United States at (800) 762-2974, outside the United States at (317) 572-3993 or fax (317) 572-4002.

Wiley also publishes its books in a variety of electronic formats. Some content that appears in print may not be available in electronic books. For more information about Wiley products, visit our web site at www.wiley.com.

Library of Congress Cataloging-in-Publication Data:

Gould, Roger L., date
  Shrink yourself : break free from emotional eating forever /
Roger Gould.
       p. cm.
  Includes bibliographical references and index.
  ISBN 978-0-470-04485-8 (cloth)
  ISBN 978-0-470-27537-5 (paper)
1. Compulsive   eating—Popular   works. 2.   Food   habits—Psychological aspects—Popular works. 3.   Weight loss—Psychological aspects—Popular works. 4.   Self-help techniques.   I. Title.
  RC552.C65G68 2007
  616.85'26—dc22

                                                              2006032487

Printed in the United States of America

10   9   8   7   6   5

To my wife, Bonnie,
who knows how to love, and to be loved

Contents

Acknowledgments

This book is derived from the MasteringFood.com program, so I want to thank my staff, who worked with me over several years to write and think through the complex logic of that program. They are Michael Vogt, Dan Marshall, and Peter Verukailen.

I want to give special thanks and acknowledgment to Hiyaguha Rachelle Cohen, who has been my constant editor on this and related projects for the last three years. She has been an invaluable second pair of eyes who helped transform the material from the online MasteringFood program into a book rich and complete with real-life stories. Her faithful renditions of my case examples and the principles of this book and her artful suggestions about making complex concepts concrete and accessible are the products of her own professional experiences as psychologist and author. This book could not have happened without her.

I want to thank my editor, Tom Miller, who immediately knew the importance of what we are hoping to do and made the key suggestion as to how this book would be best organized.

I want to thank Michelle Fiordaliso, who joined my staff late, but was here to make the final draft final, and made many important contributions along the way.

And, of course, my agent Sandra Dijkstra, for making sure these ideas became a book.

Introduction

Twenty years ago, I started working with psychotherapy outpatients who also had eating issues. When these patients told me that they had trouble controlling their weight because they ate too much, I would ask, "Why do you eat too much once you've decided not to?" You can imagine the answers I got as I pursued the question over the years. The answers ran the gamut of everything that has been reported in every self-help diet book, in every online diary, in every confessional written by the morbidly obese, the bulimic, or your average everyday overeater. "I eat because I'm ravenously hungry." "I eat because I'm bored, or lonely, or married, or single." "I eat because I pass a donut shop, or I had too much to drink, or I was at a party." "I eat because my mother cooked and I didn't want to disappoint her, or because I want to eat as much as my husband can, or I don't want to deprive myself, or I'm depressed." For years, my exploration of this question led nowhere. My patients would talk about the problem, we would understand some of the illogic behind the pattern and some of the historical connections with early family experiences, but all the explorations remained superficial. I kept on hitting brick walls. My patients went around and around in circles, telling me things like "I ate because I was angry at Joe, vowed not to do that again, but felt so guilty about eating that I just said the hell with the diet, and went on to eat as much as I wanted. I guess I'm powerless when it comes to food, just too weak to do this right."

Eventually it sank in. "I'm powerless" was the key. I was exploring the wrong question. It's not "Why do you eat?" It's "Why are you powerless?" Why, after you made a commitment to yourself to take charge of your eating, did the urge to eat become so powerful that it, or that part of you, overruled your conscious intent? There was not only an urge to eat, there was a conflict occurring between two parts of your mind fighting over who was going to control that moment when your hand moved toward the chocolate cake.

Once I had that realization, I was in familiar territory, and my understanding of the answer to the new question "Why are you powerless?" quickly grew. I saw the issues of overeating as closely aligned with those I had observed in my work developing programs for alcoholism and addiction. The alcoholic and the addict both felt they were powerless when it came to alcohol and drugs, but it was very clear that the real powerlessness was about some aspect of their life. When things went wrong, they turned to these dangerous and illegal substances, while people who struggled with their weight had found a legal, readily available tranquilizer to serve the same purpose.

I also realized that overeating issues had some relevance to the stages of life we normally go through in maturing. My book about the stages of life, *Transformations: Growth and Change in Adult Life*, was organized around one aspect of powerlessness: the question of safety. In *Shrink Yourself*, I focus on the maturation of your conscience, because it's your overly critical conscience that creates the illusion of being powerless when you're not really powerless. My training as a psychoanalyst immersed me in the complexities of this internal drama between you and your critical conscience, and that has become the main underlying theme of this book about taking charge of your weight and your life.

For decades, starting when I was the head of Outpatient and

Community Psychiatry at U.C.L.A, I've been developing computer-assisted psychotherapy programs to make therapy more affordable. About five years ago I put it all together to create an online step-by-step program that guides people through all the ways they unnecessarily conclude that they're helpless or powerless over their uncontrollable urge to eat. Several thousand people used my online program MasteringFood, which was the predecessor to the Shrink Yourself Hunger Coach (www.shrinkyourself.com). I'm writing this book to share what I've learned, and what has already worked for thousands of people.

All people, when it comes to controlling their weight, are looking for a simple or even magical solution. You don't need to go far to see that. Everywhere you look, someone is advertising a new diet, a new pill, a new exercise plan, or a new surgical solution. I wish I could offer you a simple way to remedy something you've struggled with for so long, but I can't. Instead, what I can offer you is something born out of years of experience. I've come to believe that the issue of powerlessness is the key to controlling your weight. It's the missing link. It's the reason your attempts to lose weight have failed or why your successes have only been temporary. What I'm offering isn't a simple solution but rather an interesting and proven process that will have you recover your power not only over food, but over many aspects of your life.

Why Do You Eat?

Food starts off as being not just a source of life but an expression of love. At the heart of almost every culture, hospitality is shown by feeding people. And a celebration or a time of grief wouldn't be complete without food.

Using food for reasons other than simple sustenance is a normal part of life. It becomes a problem when food becomes so closely linked with feelings that the two overlap and become one. The foundation for this starts in childhood. "When I was good, I got a cookie"; "When I fell down, I was offered food"; "On summer nights, we went to the lake to get ice cream"; "Sitting at the kitchen table eating bologna sandwiches and chips was the only time I had with my mother"; "When I misbehaved, dessert was withheld." Food was transformed from a simple source of nutrition to a reward, a diversion, a punishment, a love object, a friend. Once that happened, food became a way to control your emotions—to deal with your feelings of powerlessness. When you've installed food as a preferred way to cope, you stop developing new ways to deal with stress, your weight becomes increasingly difficult to control, and ultimately you end up reinforcing your feelings of powerlessness.

In simple terms, when something happens to bother you (such as a person ignoring you), it makes you feel bad, and you suddenly have the uncontrollable urge to eat. Then, when you eat more than you know you should, it's always followed by regret, self-hatred, and extra pounds. For many of you, the moment when something bothers you overlaps with the moment when you suddenly have the uncontrollable urge to eat. For instance, my patient Gloria, a married woman who is thirty-three years old and thirty pounds overweight, told me about an eating episode that occurred after an argument with her husband. I asked her why she chose to eat to deal with how she was feeling. She responded, "What other choice did I have?" In the next half-hour of the session, we developed six other things that she could've done instead of eating. For example, she could have taken responsibility for her part of the argument or done something to relax, like going for a walk or taking a bath, to buy herself some time to think things through and clarify her feelings. I was struck over the years by how many people were similar to Gloria. Something happened, and they felt that there wasn't any other choice but to deal with what happened by eating. They gave up because they felt powerless. By choosing food, they totally relinquished their ability to solve problems and deal with their lives in a mature and empowered way, and this naturally reinforced their experience of powerlessness. The only way to recover that power is to pause long enough to determine what other options you have besides eating when something in life troubles you. Even though it may not be obvious that something happened that bothered you, if you suddenly find yourself starving when you know you've just eaten, you can logically suspect that you've been emotionally triggered in some way.

Extensive research has shown that you're not really starving in those moments. It's almost always emotional hunger that drives you: a fight with a spouse, an uncomfortable work situation, a lull in your workday, a needy parent or child, your life, your future, your past. It's something that sets off a brief episode of powerlessness.

This book is really about finding the space between when something has affected you and your sudden urge to eat (which is not real hunger), and then exploring what goes on in your mind when you have that uncontrollable urge. Up until now, the emotions and issues that fuel the urge to eat have been operating behind the scenes, sabotaging all of your good intentions.

Who Will Benefit from *Shrink Yourself*?

This book will benefit anyone who feels that they have an unhealthy relationship with food. Some people aren't even overweight and yet their thoughts are still consumed with what they're going to eat and food is still the way they manage their emotions and cope with stress. Focusing on food distracts them from dealing with the other real issues in their lives. This book is for anyone who has too often used food to deal with the challenges and struggles of life.

Food, when used to make you feel better, actually impedes your ability to be informed by your feelings, to complete your emotional maturation, and to have the fulfilling life that you dream about. Once we bring the spotlight back to the real issues and take the focus away from food and weight, you'll begin to see who you really are, what you really want, and how to get it. Once you do this, you'll become like the person in love, or the child at play who doesn't want to come in for dinner, or the artist in the studio so fixated on creation that he forgets to eat. You will have recovered your power.

If you're ready to explore why losing weight has been so difficult for so long so that you can finally be free of your food addiction forever, this book is for you.

How Does the Book Work?

Once I began to explore the question of powerlessness as related to weight, I realized that powerlessness over the urge to eat was simply a superficial layer of powerlessness. It actually covered up for five other ways that people felt powerless in their lives. People feel powerless when they doubt themselves, when they feel frustrated, when they feel vulnerable or unsafe, when they feel rebellious or angry, and when they feel empty. I call these five areas the *five layers of powerlessness*, which we'll explore throughout this book. As you explore each of these layers, you'll delve more deeply into your psyche and develop a more mature and clear view of who you are and who you are becoming.

When a person crosses over the line between food as a source of life and food as a source of comfort, all these layers compound one another and food becomes a psychological thing instead of a biological necessity. People can usually identify when in their lives this happened. Perhaps it was during a difficult transition: a divorce, a move, or a change of schools. But whenever it happened, they have perpetuated the pattern and they can't see their way out. This book will help you peel away the layers and finally be free of this pattern.

In this first part of the book, you'll learn about these five layers and how they've been specifically affecting your life. Then, in part two, you'll have sessions that, similar to being in a private session with me or participating in my twelve-week program, will provide you with the necessary exercises to have you arrive at the insights and understanding you need to achieve real change.

Together we'll peel away the layers as you go on the *Shrink Yourself* journey, and I'll work with you through the exercises in this book to free the real you hiding inside your body.

We'll look at why, after so many efforts to be free of an addiction to food, you're still at a place where you feel utterly defeated. Together we'll begin again—this time with a renewed sense of hope and my expertise and partnership. As you strip away each of the layers of powerlessness, your dependence on food will diminish until your powerful self finally emerges.

PART ONE

The Learning Sessions

1

Emotional Eating 101

*I've been on a constant diet for the last two decades. I've
lost a total of 789 pounds. By all accounts, I should be
hanging from a charm bracelet.—Erma Bombeck*

Take any moment in time, focus the camera lens on your neighborhood, and look closely. You'll find dozens of people—maybe even
hundreds or thousands—breaking their diets no matter when you
check. Every one of those well-intentioned dieters woke up in the
morning determined to stick to an eating plan, but by afternoon had
one hand on a piece of chocolate and the other on their forehead,
wondering why, why on earth they had no willpower. In fact, you
might be one of those people.

It's no secret that extra pounds can shorten your life. Studies
show that up to 83 percent of diabetes, hypertension, and heart disease can be prevented by proper diet and exercise. Obesity can
diminish your energy level, interfere with social success, and even
reduce earnings, as a recent study that appeared in the *Los Angeles
Times* showed. The study measured overall wealth at age thirty-nine

for 2,000 people who had been followed since adolescence. Those with a normal weight had twice as much accumulated wealth.

So why can't you reach your weight goals, knowing these things?

As I said in the Introduction, you have installed food as a psychological coping mechanism in addition to being a source of nutrition.

My patient Allison recently told me, "My dependence on food started as a preteen. If I came home sad, my mother told me, 'Eat, it'll make you feel better.' I didn't have weight problems very early on in life but I was pushed to eat, eat. As a teenager, food became my friend.

"One day when I was sixteen, I found out that my boyfriend had cheated on me with this bitchy girl, Linda. I remember crying on the couch and my mom making me a huge ice cream sundae and spoon-feeding it to me. And yes, if you can believe it, I still want ice cream now whenever I feel blue. When my divorce from Tad became final last month, I went right out to Cold Stone Creamery. I know I eat to avoid emotions."

Using food to deal with emotions as Linda did is called *emotional eating*. A study I conducted of 17,000 failed dieters showed that virtually all of them relapsed because of emotional issues, mostly related to self-esteem or emotional hurt. They were doing really well on their diets, and then their husband started having an affair, or they lost their job, or a parent got sick. Perhaps you had a similar kind of thing trip up your diet efforts in the past.

One thing I've learned is that attacking emotional hunger by counting calories is almost like trying to run a marathon while lying on your couch. It just doesn't make any sense. You need to go deep within to control emotional hunger, because as real as the hunger feels, it originates in your mind, not in your belly.

Roxy, a forty-five-year-old mother of three, reported that she ate a whole box of donuts after a frustrating afternoon at the mall with her sixteen-year-old daughter. She said to me, "I was so mad at her, what else could I do?" This very intelligent woman couldn't think of even one other option, in spite of my prompting and questioning.

Her pattern of stuffing down feelings by stuffing in food was so deeply ingrained in her mind that it short-circuited her common sense. Roxy had lost her ability to think clearly and constructively about a charged emotional issue, another indication of emotional eating. She didn't need a box of donuts to satisfy her physical hunger, but she thought she did. She thought donuts were the only way to dial down her anger and frustration and to rid herself of angry thoughts toward her daughter.

Roxy and Allison have a few things in common.

1. They overate to suppress feelings.
2. They chose comfort food (not broccoli) and felt guilty about it.
3. They short-circuited their best problem-solving abilities.

These three behaviors describe emotional eating in a nutshell.

Let's start with a simple quiz to determine if you are in fact an emotional eater, someone who uses food to cope with life.

Are You an Emotional Eater?

To find out if you're an emotional eater, answer the following seven questions.

The last time you ate too much:

1. Did you notice your hunger coming on fast, or did it grow gradually?
2. When you got hungry, did you feel an almost desperate need to eat something right away?
3. When you ate, did you pay attention to what went in your mouth, or did you just stuff it in?
4. When you got hungry, would any nutritious food have sufficed, or did you need a certain type of food or treat to satisfy yourself?

5. Did you feel guilty after you ate?

6. Did you eat when you were emotionally upset or experiencing feelings of "emptiness"?

7. Did you stuff in the food very quickly?

Let's see how you did.

1. Emotional hunger comes on suddenly, while physical hunger develops slowly. Physical hunger begins with a tummy rumble, then it becomes a stronger grumble, and finally it evolves into hunger pangs, but it's a slow process, very different from emotional hunger, which has a sudden, dramatic onset.

2. Unlike physical hunger, emotional hunger demands food immediately, and it wants immediate satisfaction. Physical hunger, on the other hand, will wait for food.

3. A difference between physical and emotional hunger involves mindfulness. To satisfy physical hunger, you normally make a deliberate choice about what you consume, and you maintain awareness of what you eat. You notice how much you put in your mouth so that you can stop when you're full. Emotional hunger, in contrast, rarely notices what's being eaten. If you have emotional hunger, you'll want more food even after you're stuffed.

4. Emotional hunger often demands particular foods in order to be fulfilled. If you're physically hungry, even carrots will look delicious. If you're emotionally hungry, however, only cake or ice cream or your particular preferred indulgence will seem appealing.

5. Emotional hunger often results in guilt or promises to do better next time. Physical hunger has no guilt attached to it, because you know you ate in order to maintain health and energy.

6. Emotional hunger results from some emotional trigger. Physical hunger results from a physiological need.

7. When you are feeding physical hunger, you can eat your food and savor each bite, but when you eat to fulfill emotional hunger you stuff the food in. All of a sudden you look down and the whole pint of ice cream is gone.

The Real Reason You're So Hungry— Phantom Hunger

When I buy cookies I eat just four and throw the rest away. But first I spray them with Raid so I won't dig them out of the garbage later. Be careful, though, because that Raid really doesn't taste that bad.—*Janette Barber*

Did your answers to the seven questions above reveal that you might be an emotional eater? Did you discover that you've been confusing emotional hunger with real, biological hunger? If so, the first question becomes—why?

You eat when you aren't really hungry because you have two stomachs—one real, the other phantom. The hunger in your belly signals you when your system has a biological requirement for food. If that was the only signal of hunger you received, you'd be thin. It's the phantom stomach that causes the problems. The phantom stomach sends out a signal demanding food when unruly emotions and unsolved personal agendas start pushing themselves into awareness and you feel compelled to eat, or more accurately to stuff yourself and shut the feelings up. Phantom hunger has such power that it drives you to almost any lengths to satisfy it. You'll drive to a convenience store in the middle of the night for snacks; you'll steal your child's Halloween candy when she's asleep; you'll sneak and hide food.

My patient Danielle described an episode of phantom hunger on a typical weekend: "The minute my husband left the house to play golf I found myself getting 'hungry' when I knew I wasn't. I tried to put eating off: I took the dog for a walk, I went in the hot tub . . . but the entire time I only thought of what I could be making, what I could be eating. I checked the fridge I don't know how many times, and then the pantry . . . then the fridge. Three cookies, some spoon-fuls of ice cream, slices of cheese, a handful of cashews, five more cookies, the rest of the pack. Then I sat in front of the TV and wham—I'm 'hungry' again. Every time the show stopped and a com-mercial came on, I wanted something else to eat."

Danielle didn't know what to do with herself when she was alone. Sound familiar, or do you have other triggers that drive you to the cupboard? All emotional eaters have particular issues they want to avoid facing, and when those issues arise, the phantom belly growls with insistent urgency and suddenly you find yourself pow-erless over the urge to eat.

What Triggers Your Phantom Hunger?

There are two categories of things that trigger phantom hunger. The first includes situations, places, or events. Perhaps you overeat when you have to attend staff meetings at your pathetic job, or when you go to family functions. For some people, it's funerals or restaurants or sports events. For others, it's a boring day at work.

The second category that triggers phantom hunger includes people. For you, it's probably a specific person—your boss, parent, spouse, or child—who triggers you to overeat. They may trigger you with a glance, a word, or even with their silence, but whatever it is, when you're around them, you're sure to overeat.

My patient Bonnie eats when she has a deadline at work. Last month, when she had a grant proposal due, she ate two large bags of chips in one day and drank four cans of soda; the next day, she had five candy bars. She gained eleven pounds in one month.

Florence, on the other hand, deals well with work pressure, but she binges late at night when her husband, Barney, doesn't come home. "I feel like I have no control," she tells me. "I get so anxious, and all I can think about is having some cake. It's always something sweet I want, and starchy, like cake or cookies or a scone. I almost get the shakes, and then I eat, and then I want something else, just to fight off the anxiety."

In other words, phantom hunger is the hunger that's created when a person feels uncomfortable.

How You Originally Got Hooked on Food

If you do have an emotional eating pattern, you might wonder where it came from. Did you become an emotional eater because you have extraordinary problems or some genetic coding gone awry? Probably not. Emotional eating is the norm at birth for all of us. When a mother feeds her baby, the baby stops crying because food soothes. Babies equate the mother's milk with survival, love, and peace of mind. When babies don't get mother's milk, they may settle for a substitute—a bottle or a pacifier, for instance. The pacifier has no warmth, taste, or nutritional value, but it's close enough to that primal experience to soothe the infant. It's natural for infants to continuously seek comfort from the mother's soothing presence, and easy enough, later in life, to make food the substitute pathway back to that comforting state of mind.

The first, and primal, regulator of your mood was your mother. If your needs for food and comfort were met, then you will often equate that comfort on some level with food. And if you were neglected in some way by your caregivers, food and love will be linked and you'll find yourself craving food when what you really want is love.

As you grew up you had to learn to regulate your own moods and handle stressful situations, away from your mother, without the immediacy of food or her love. You had to develop the mental skill to handle your interior life as an autonomous being. If you still use food as an artificial quick switch to stop feeling bad and start feeling good, you've not yet completed this essential task of human development. You want to be independent, but perhaps you also fear or resist it. You'll learn more about this ambivalence later in this book.

Although decades have passed since infancy, you still have a sense-memory left over from this buried part of your past, so that even now, eating actually changes the state of your mind, at least temporarily. When you feel anxious, eating "compresses" the anxiety, almost as if it's dialing down the volume. Overeating actually works. It soothes you in times of distress, and that's the dilemma. But as you know, the comfort doesn't last for long, because once the food is finished, the self-hatred starts.

You probably adopted food as a method to cope with uncomfortable feelings at some point in your development, when in an effort to return to the safety of infancy, you started overeating. Perhaps it was when your parents separated, or when you changed schools, or when you came home after school to an empty house, or when you went off to college, or had your first child.

For Marcia, overeating started after her family moved. "I was about eleven years old," she says. "I had just moved from the Bronx in New York to Queens, and I did not have any new friends. I would tell my parents I needed like four dollars for this special typing paper—and would go to the little grocery store and buy Twinkies, Wise potato chips, and as many other snacks as I could afford and hide them in my backpack. I would binge on cake or cookies my mother would bake and lie, saying I needed to bring them to school. I was missing some sort of attention and my old friends, I imagine, at the time it started. But I just got fat, without getting friends."

Cocaine addicts keep using cocaine because they long for the feeling of their first high, but it's something they'll never be able to get, just like Marcia couldn't go home again by eating ice cream and cake. You can't return to the comfort of infancy no matter how much food you eat.

Some of my patients say that eating puts them into a bubble where all their worries seem to disappear, much like the state that babies experience when they nurse. Others tell me that eating makes them feel insulated and protected instead of vulnerable and raw, which is like being held close to your mother's chest. You use food, whether consciously or unconsciously, to numb the mind so you don't have to deal with issues you'd rather not confront. I call the altered state of mind where food transports us a "food trance," something I'll expand upon later. It's a very important factor in the story of compulsive eating.

If you overeat when you feel distress in order to change your state of mind, then food has become your substitute for that mother–child bliss. Certainly, when you go to the vending machine when you just can't deal with your workday you aren't thinking about cuddling with Mom, but that's the unconscious origin of the urge to overeat, and it's as primal as can be. In psychological terms, food has become a love object. Separating you from your food is like yanking the child out of the arms of her mother; destroying your private, secret sanctuary; and exposing you to the unending turmoil of life. No wonder you hold onto your emotional eating pattern with such tenacity—the alternative is too frightening. It makes perfect sense!

Why Is Emotional Eating So Hard to Stop?

Inside some of us is a thin person struggling to get out, but they can usually be sedated with a few pieces of chocolate cake.
—*Anonymous*

Basically, all diet plans and fitness programs advise you to just cut back or choose what you eat according to some logical plan. These strategies imply that you can consciously control your eating habits, choose alfalfa sprouts instead of ice cream, and deal with life's problems straight on. For emotional eaters, however, this simply isn't possible; the urge to eat is too strong. Food has become a psychological tool, a way to avoid feelings that are too intense or anxiety-provoking. If you haven't learned how to cope with your life and your emotions in a way that doesn't include food, you will not be able to adhere to any diet plan for very long. While things are going smoothly in your life you may be able to stick to your diet, but when life presents a challenge you'll inevitably turn back to your old faithful fix, food.

Using food to deal with feelings, however, creates a vicious cycle. Food lets you avoid your problems or what's bothering you for a while, but when problems are left unattended they grow in intensity. This makes you stuff yourself and then you're filled with guilt on top of your original problem, and the cycle spirals out of control because then you need food to deal with the guilt as well as the original problem. Sure, food can serve as a fabulous quick fix, it can bring immediate relief and pleasure, but it doesn't take long to see that one cookie doesn't do it. You end up needing more and more to fill up the emptiness from living an unexamined life.

Emotional eaters have struggled with this vicious cycle for years in some cases or even decades. It's so difficult to change the cycle because simply recognizing it doesn't help, nor does willpower. In order to change this deeply entrenched pattern, you have to go deep below the surface to new places never before explored. You need to analyze what's happening in your life—you need to address that which you're trying to avoid by eating, and arrive at a new response. That is the only way to break the cycle. That's what we're going to do together.

Powerlessness

After working with thousands of emotional eaters, I've been able to decode the secret of overeating and break it down to reveal some basic truths. You think the main thing you're struggling with is feeling powerless over your uncontrollable urge to eat. However, years of experience have proved to me that that sense of powerlessness over food, although deeply agonizing, is really a cover-up, and the consequence, of a deeper experience of powerlessness.

1. You feel powerless about how to deal with your self-doubts.
2. You feel powerless about how to get real satisfaction in life.

3. You feel powerless to insure your own safety.

4. You feel powerless to appropriately assert your independence.

5. You feel powerless to fill yourself up when you feel empty inside.

You eat when you feel powerless in one or more of these five ways, because the experience of powerlessness is almost instantaneously transformed into the uncontrollable urge to eat. This fact is the cornerstone of everything that follows in this book.

We'll teach you how to overcome these five experiences of powerlessness by focusing on the fact that you are not really powerless, but instead are needlessly giving away the power you do have over control of yourself and your life. Once you realize that, your urge to eat will be controllable, and you'll reclaim your power in your relationship to food and increase your power in all the areas of your life

Compulsion versus Motivation

In one Native American folk tale, a grandfather explains to his grandson that he has two wolves inside him. One wolf fills him with hope and reminds him how wonderful his life is, and the other fills him with doubt and convinces him that nothing is worth the effort. The grandson asks, concerned for his grandfather, "Which wolf will win?" The grandfather replies, "Whichever one I feed."

The two wolves inside you are your positive motivations to lose weight versus your experience of powerlessness that leads to the uncontrollable urge to eat, and the overeating camp usually wins. Every time you overeat because you are *feeling* powerless, you reinforce your erroneous belief that you *are* powerless. You feed the wrong wolf.

No matter how hard you try to diet, no matter how sincere your promise to give up certain foods, you can't stop overeating for very long. When you do, you feel empty or anxious. Feelings of depression and boredom begin to creep in. As long as you remain unaware of the experience of powerlessness and how it's instantaneously transformed into the uncontrollable urge to eat, you can't change it.

Once you begin to look at the fact that overeating has served you in some way, you may be ready to see that the fact that you haven't been able to lose the weight you want has nothing to do with your willpower, and it isn't because you haven't found the right diet or the magic solution, either. You haven't been able to lose the weight you want because eating has become an automatic soothing response to the stresses in your life.

My goal is to help you become mindful, conscious, observant, and awake in order to find the pause between when you have one of the five experiences of powerlessness and when you begin to overeat. It's only in that space that you can begin to change your emotional eating pattern. Because it happens so quickly, you are not even aware at this point that you are making a decision. But you are, so in each chapter and in each session we are going to try to slow the process down by looking at the gap between the experience of powerlessness and the uncontrollable urge to eat in great detail. That will give you the opportunity to make a different decision.

Diets Fail Because of Emotional Eating

Diets don't work—for you or for anyone. Of course, eventually you'll have to adhere to a sensible eating plan and a regular exercise routine, but first you must focus on what specifically makes you feel powerless in your life, especially in relation to food.

You may be hopeful now at the start of this journey, but I suspect that you're also skeptical about ultimate success. Your gut may be saying to you, "Can something as deep and as strong as my emotional eating pattern really be changed?"

The answer is "yes"; thousands of people have already gone through the Shrink Yourself program online and have been able to reclaim their power and make dramatic changes in their relationship with food, reversing patterns that had been there for decades. Some of the members of Shrink Yourself have said, "I learned things that I tried to hide from myself and your program found all of them. I learned I don't need to let food and eating rule and ruin me and have already lost sixteen pounds," or "The program was a great way to mirror back behaviors, motivations, and habits that were not serving me well. It gave me a deeper understanding of how destructive these were to my health and happiness—my focus is finally on me and not food"; and finally, "The program showed me how to see what was really bothering me in my life. Once I started to address those things and make changes, the fat just became a useless blanket I was hiding beneath."

But this place of skepticism is where everyone who has attained lifelong weight loss has to start. Once you get past that, we'll be ready to look at what has kept you stuck in the same vicious cycle for so long.

You see, the diet industry assumes that because you're desperate to lose weight, you'll have enough positive motivation to stick to the program and succeed. As you've discovered, eating generates immediate rewards, whereas the rewards you get from dieting won't be realized for weeks, months, or, for some, years. Future benefits versus the immediate compulsion to eat: that's the formula for yo-yo dieting. Positive motivation alone simply can't overcome the desire for the immediate payoff that propels you to eat the things you know you shouldn't.

I saw this fact clearly demonstrated when I consulted at the Pritikin Institute in Santa Monica, California, where clients paid $10,000 a month to take part in a controlled diet and exercise program. Although the tuition for the program far exceeded the cost of attending the most expensive private university in America, I frequently found participants sneaking out for hamburgers and french fries at a corner stand. These were all highly motivated people sent to Pritikin by their doctors because of serious, life-threatening health problems, but positive motivation clearly wasn't enough to help them resist phantom hunger.

One recent study showed that 33 percent of overweight women said they would trade 5 percent of their remaining lifetime for just ten pounds of permanent fat loss. With that level of desperation, you would expect these women to succeed in dropping pounds, but they don't succeed, so again, you see that negative motivation easily overpowers even the most positive motivation in the weight-loss arena. The desire to hold onto the comforts of emotional eating can be a powerful force indeed—far more powerful than the desire to shed the belly.

Don't be discouraged if you recognize how much you now love and depend on food—if you fear that you won't be able to function if you stop overeating. It's the place where everyone must start. All you need is a good therapist to take you on a healing journey.

SHRINK YOURSELF SESSION NOTES
Emotional Eating

- You've defined yourself as an emotional eater.
- You're beginning to look at the differences between phantom hunger and physical hunger.
- You're starting to see glimpses of how you began using food as a source of comfort or a reward.
- You know the secret to overeating is not your lack of willpower but your experience of powerlessness.
- You have to remember that in the gap between powerlessness and the uncontrollable urge to eat, you are making a decision that can be changed.
- You'll have to rid yourself of denial in order to do the learning work that will free you from your food addiction.

2

Food, the Over-the-Counter Tranquilizer

Christine, a forty-year-old patient of mine, had just moved back to Los Angeles from Alabama. While she was living in the South she gained fifty pounds. It wasn't just the down-home cooking, it was being in an abusive relationship and then living alone in an unsafe neighborhood. She was already ashamed about her weight when she moved back home to L.A.—after all she used to be a model— but she was determined to have a fresh start. This time, she was going to get what she deserved from her job and from her relation- ships. She was going to do everything right from day one. When she was offered a job the first week back, she didn't negotiate a high enough salary for herself. She got off the phone feeling defeated, her chance to have a clean slate ruined, just like when you blow your diet and you figure why bother for the rest of the day. She didn't realize that she was feeling all of these things, though; she just hung up the phone and suddenly felt hungry.

In the last chapter we defined emotional eating as using food to deal with your experience of powerlessness over the struggles and stresses of life. We established that something always triggers you to overeat, perhaps some friction with someone or an emotionally relevant event in your life. Now let's look deeper. It's not the person or the event per se that sets you off, but how those things made you feel. At first you may not even know how you feel. As you work on shrinking yourself, you'll observe the places you're at or the people you're around when you tend to overeat. Then you'll pay close attention to what feelings come up for you around those people or situations.

Marjorie is thirty-eight years old and is married with two children. She had twenty-five pounds to lose after her first child was born and now she has forty pounds to lose after her second child. She said, "I've started to notice that every time I go to my mother-in-law's house, even though I'm not hungry, I go right toward food. I use the food like a weapon, even though I'm only hurting myself, not my mother-in-law, who triggered the emotion."

Simply identifying the times when you overeat is a huge first step. Why is it a huge step? It's a huge step because then things start to come into focus. You'll be putting a spotlight on something, and that will allow you to begin to analyze it. Inevitably, you'll have to confront the bad feelings that, up until now, you've been trying to get rid of by eating.

Let's face it: there isn't anyone who welcomes bad feelings. We look to do something with them—wish them away, take a nap, go for a jog, talk to a friend, distract ourselves with television or a book, have a drink, smoke a cigarette, have sex, or eat a snack. Ideally you can get to a point where bad feelings are like bad weather—you know they'll pass, and just like when you know it's going to rain so you bring your umbrella, you know what you need to get through them. If you haven't yet arrived at this place of acceptance where even bad feelings are a part of you to include rather than to banish, then food will remain your preferred method of medicating yourself.

Food Protects You from Bad Feelings

Why has food become the thing that you consistently turn to when feelings triggered by people or events feel unbearable? Food serves two very effective purposes. First, it helps you avoid feelings. I call the desire to avoid emotions the "feeling phobia." Also, food gives you a way to replace bad feelings with the pleasurable experience of eating. I call the pleasurable experience that food provides the "food trance." In short, eating protects you from the feelings that you don't want to feel.

If your feelings open the door to your interior world, then eating slams the door shut. It keeps you functioning on a surface level, and although you're feeling powerless to control what and how much you eat, at least you don't have to focus on the deeper things that really make you feel powerless (including failed relationships, unsatisfying careers, and difficult children). Remember Christine from the beginning of this chapter? Not handling her job opportunity perfectly gave Christine a flood of bad feelings: disappointment, fear that her new start was already ruined, and anger at herself. By eating, she got to avoid confronting all those feelings.

Many people report to me that as they're approaching their goal weight they often sabotage themselves and all of their efforts. They wonder why that is. It doesn't seem to make any sense. In fact, you may be able to relate to that experience. The answer, time and again, proves to be simple: if you didn't have your weight to think about you might have to think about what's really bothering you, and that's very frightening. It's frightening because I know that you feel powerless to change the things that really bother you. You've made what I call the "unexamined powerlessness conclusion." It's a conclusion that you're powerless over your feelings and the circumstances in your life that the feelings point toward, so you might as well eat.

Food Reinforces Your Feelings of Powerlessness

We talked about how eating takes you to an earlier place in your development, predominantly because as infants and children, food was often associated with comfort and love. However, childhood is also associated with powerlessness. As a child, you were in fact powerless. You could be mistreated, you couldn't control your impulses, you were subject to abandonment, you were dependent on others to protect and nurture you. Although food provides you with some of the comfort of infancy by taking you back to that state of mind, when you use food this way, you're reverting back to a childish way of dealing with the world. And that reminds you of the powerless feeling of being a child. You're an adult now and you have choices: you can be the powerful agent of your own life by facing your feelings and hearing what they have to say to you, or you can continue eating to cope with emotions, knowing that it actually keeps you stuck in childhood, a place where you were in fact powerless. Facing your feelings makes you an adult, the only place where you have the possibility to finally be powerful.

For emotional eaters like yourself, you can't see the forest for the trees. In the moment when feelings have been triggered and an unexamined powerlessness conclusion has been made, eating feels like a life-or-death decision. When you distract yourself with food, it's not an apple or a simple cookie. It tends to be large quantities of food, typically unhealthy foods, and the foods are eaten in a voracious, aggressive way—more like stuffing than eating. By the time the eating frenzy has ended, the bad feelings have vanished, but they aren't really gone. They're just buried under food, almost like lost files on a hard drive—they exist somewhere but are temporarily irretrievable. You're addicted to the escape that the food provides you more than to the food itself.

The Feeling Phobia

"Comfort me with apples: for I am sick with love."—Song of Solomon 2:5

Alice, a thirty-year-old online member who reports feeling addicted to food, is successful at her job. She hasn't found a satisfying relationship yet, and when she comes home after work she often feels lonely. She said, "It gets too quiet if I'm not chewing."

Why, exactly, do you eat to cope with uncomfortable feelings? Why do you eat in order to avoid dealing with the sensations aroused by strong emotions? Are you like a patient of mine who said, "I stuff my mouth with food when I'm angry because I'm afraid I might bite someone"?

What is it about emotion that triggers overeating? Why wouldn't you want to just face your anger, experience it, get over it, instead of choking down your feelings? What's so terrible about emotion anyway? That's the root question. Once you understand why you interrupt your negative feelings rather than let them flow to their natural outcome, you can make a rational decision about whether it makes more sense to deal with those feelings or to eat. Right now, it's automatic; you don't really have a choice to make.

No one likes feeling angry, lonely, bored, or sad. But most emotional eaters have more than a simple dislike of these feelings, they have an allergic reaction to them. In fact, I believe that most emotional eaters have what I call a "feeling phobia." This phobia makes you avoid negative emotions at any cost because you're overly frightened of what your feelings mean and where they might lead you. For example, I've heard patients say that if they didn't eat they would cry for days. But most people who have had a good cry know that once you stop clenching your throat and quivering your lip and let the tears come, you feel much lighter. You've probably been holding your feelings in for so long that you don't believe you can deal with them. This is normal.

Feelings are the doorway you need to pass through. You have to stop eating mindlessly and automatically when unpleasant feelings arise so that you can draw on your interior wisdom.

We're meaning-hungry creatures. We make everything mean something. When we come home at the end of our busy days we look at our e-mail in box or our answering machine, and if there are no messages we make that mean something. If there are many messages we make that mean something, too. Sometimes we attribute off-base meaning to things in our lives. Most often we misinterpret our feelings in a way that confirms that we're not as worthy as we'd like to be, that makes us believe we're more powerless than we actually are. These misinterpretations turn up the volume on simple emotions.

You typically interpret the actions of others and events in your life and even the feelings you're having in a particular way, a way that leaves you feeling bad. Have you ever noticed that when you're watching someone else's child and that child misbehaves, you can address their behavior calmly? However, when your own child exhibits the same behavior you find yourself beet red and screaming. Have you ever wondered why that is? It's because when your child misbehaves you make his behavior mean something about the future of your child (if he keeps behaving like this he's destined to be a serial killer) or you make it mean something about you (I would never have been allowed to get away with crap like this). It's the interpretation that makes the feeling so intense.

Catastrophe Predictions

Feelings are like weather. They're all necessary. Living in Southern California, I have seen how a slight drizzle can almost shut the city down. People are not accustomed to dealing with rain, and so they panic when it happens. The rain is not really the problem. It's what they say about the rain that scares them (it will be dangerous to drive, there will be more traffic; my kids will have to play inside now). And so it is the same with your feelings. The feelings themselves are not problematic; it's normal and healthy to have all kinds of different feelings. Where we get stuck and panicked is when we interpret what those feelings mean. There's a specific way in which you misinterpret your feelings and experiences that I call "catastrophe predictions." You misinterpret things in a way that paints a very vivid portrait of how terrible things are going to turn out. Catastrophe predictions are doomsday thoughts that are, in fact, not true. They reflect the worst that your brain imagines is possible.

Instead of experiencing sadness, you see yourself being depressed forever. Instead of feeling loneliness, you see yourself as a seventy-year-old spinster with sixteen cats. Instead of dealing with simple anger, you're afraid you'll hurt someone.

Norma is a thirty-six-year-old mother of three. Every day at 4:30 P.M., she starts to count the hours until her husband will get home. She gets so overwhelmed and it feels as if she'll never get any relief from the laundry, the kids fighting, and her mother, who, recently widowed, is dating on a regular basis and wants Norma to be her confidante about her new sexual endeavors. The day feels endless, Norma feels totally alone, and it's during those hours that she finds herself bingeing on all of the kids' snacks. By the time her husband gets home, she's disgusted with herself.

When Norma starts to have the catastrophe prediction that she'll never get any relief, instead of just acknowledging how tired she is by 4:30 and doing something to make that time of day easier, she feels powerless and the uncontrollable urge to eat shows up.

As you shrink yourself by doing the exercises in part two, Session 2, you'll have to identify the catastrophe predictions you've been attaching to your feelings, and that will help you see why they've grown so out of proportion and subsequently why you're so afraid of them.

When you are afraid to stay with and explore your feelings, you have already come to the conclusion that you are defeated in some way. Your feelings are leading to a deeper experience of powerlessness, and that's where you don't want to go. As you know, the emotional eating pattern gets triggered like a knee-jerk reaction. Something happens, you make a misinterpretation—perhaps a catastrophe prediction—and you arrive at a powerlessness conclusion, all in the blink of an eye. When you come to the place where you're feeling powerless for just a moment, you believe on some level that eating is the only option that you really have to make yourself feel better, and that otherwise that moment will become an eternity.

I listed the several types of powerlessness conclusions that you might have experienced in the last chapter, and will go into them in greater detail in the remaining chapters, but for now let's look at them a bit more closely so that you can get some clarity on what's really going on for you when you make the decision to overeat despite your commitment to control your weight.

Powerlessness Conclusions

Conclusion # 1: Your Self-Doubt Layer   Someone asks you to do something at work that you don't know how to do. You come to the powerless conclusion that you're stupid. To feel this way is so devastating, but you don't have to go to the vending machine and eat to avoid feeling stupid. *In part two, I'll show you how to talk back to your inner critic and erase the idea that the real you is stupid.*

Conclusion # 2: Your Reward/Frustration Layer   You go on your eighteenth date from Match.com. No one feels right despite all the hope you have going into each date. You come to the conclusion that you're defeated and there's nothing you can do about it. The search for a good mate can be disappointing, but you don't have to deal with it by stopping at a fast food restaurant on your way home. *In part two, I'll show you how to work on your relationships.*

Conclusion # 3: Your Safety Layer   You were molested as a child. You come to the conclusion that you're unsafe and can't protect yourself. The trauma and pain you're feeling are real, but extra layers of fat can't change what happened to you and won't protect you from anything. *In part two, I'll show you how to create real safety by dealing with real issues.*

Conclusion # 4: Your Rebellion Layer   You're angry at your kids for never listening. You come to the conclusion that eating is better than expressing how you really feel. You're afraid that if you express how angry you are at them you'll scream uncontrollably or maybe even hit them. Anger can in fact be a frightening emotion to deal with. *In part two, I'll show you the difference between childish defiance and mature assertion.*

Conclusion # 5: Your Emptiness Layer   You almost never have plans at night. When you're alone you feel empty inside and can't experience fulfillment. You come to the conclusion that food is the only thing that can fill you up. *Being alone can be really overwhelming, but in part two, I'll start you on a pathway to being able to fulfill yourself.*

The Food Trance

Now you've seen how your feelings get so inflated that you can't think of facing them. You can understand why up until now you've wanted an escape from whatever you were experiencing—to avoid your own tendency to amp up your emotions until you feel utterly devastated, and on the brink of disaster. You've been retreating into the food trance, which feels like a safe place, a bubble, a zone where you feel nurtured, loved, free from responsibility. The food trance is a place to find rest from bad feelings—it's the place where the bad feelings are actually transformed momentarily into the pleasure of eating. The food trance is an escape. It sure beats the alternative hell of suffering through your own overblown emotions—or so it seems to you at the time.

Many of my patients over the years have described what they gain from retreating into the food trance. Maybe you'll recognize yourself in some of their comments:

Rebecca is a thirty-eight-year-old stay-at-home mom. She weighs 175 pounds and is 5'1". "Food is faithful, it's always there, always works. My husband says I make love to Kit Kat bars and he's right. I eat them methodically. It's really kind of gross but I do it each time, and every time it puts me in a trance. The short-term benefit is that for a few moments it is just me and the chocolate. My mind concentrates on the method of eating it, the taste, the texture, the sensation that doesn't allow for other thoughts or interruptions. I'm totally out of it and then when it's over it's always the same letdown—guilt and remorse."

Ellen is a single thirty-two-year-old teacher. She weighs 142 pounds and is 5'6". "Being in the food trance is very powerful. I love sweets! I have always been a slow eater, so everything I eat, I fully enjoy. When I am in a trance I savor every bite and enjoy every different flavor explosion that is happening in my mouth. All the textures dancing in my mouth provide a perfect escape for the moment. When I am concentrating on what I am eating, I don't have to deal with my emotions, but once I am done eating I am ashamed."

Lena is a sixty-three-year-old retired advertising executive. She is 5'5" and weighs 280 pounds. "The 'food trance' for me is where no one or nothing can bother you or invade you. It provides a 'numbness' to everything going on around you. I can escape, if even for a few moments. Everything is great until I come back and then the guilt sets in."

Addy is a twenty-four-year-old college student. She is 5'4" and weighs 115 pounds. "When I'm in the food trance, I stuff as much food as I can into my mouth. All of my energy goes into getting as much food as possible and eating it as fast as I can."

Reading through these comments, you probably observed that no matter how much weight the speakers have to lose, or even if they don't have weight to lose, food has become an escape. They enjoyed the food trance while they were in it, but as you saw, it was always followed by guilt and regret and, of course, extra pounds.

If food really does make you happy and contented, even if only temporarily, what a powerful narcotic it becomes. To resist it, you need to get the entire picture, to see the end of the pattern, in the way a junkie needs to see that the fast high leads to a future of overdosing, infection, poverty, crime, and so on. In the case of food compulsion, you need to see not only the weight you'll gain by eating too much—because that clearly hasn't been enough to stop you in the past—but also to understand how covering up emotions with food sets you back psychically, spiritually, and effectually.

Your feelings aren't there to make you miserable. Rather, emotions provide you with information about your interior life. Wrapped inside your feelings are messages you need to hear. Because of the catastrophe predictions you attach to emotions, you fear staying with your feelings long enough to hear yourself.

Even a seemingly innocuous feeling like boredom has something important to tell you. Your boredom might be signaling you to do what really interests you instead of what you believe you *should* do, or telling you that you miss someone or something. Boredom tells you that you hunger for a greater degree of life satisfaction than you now have, and if you listen to that boredom, it can pinch you into action so that you'll get off the recliner and start going after your dream.

You can't ignore your emotional signals—whether major or seemingly trivial—or your life will remain stuck. And if you remain stuck, you invite depression and anxiety to flourish. Of course, depression and anxiety provoke you to eat more to suppress those unwanted feelings, and the vicious cycle continues until all you know is that as soon as you feel bad, you have to eat something fast. Eventually this mechanism becomes so efficient and automatic that you aren't even aware that you feel bad. All you feel is an unrelenting pressure to eat.

Food grants you a little time-out from your life, but the time-out ends and the problems are still there. Wanting a time-out when feelings become too intense is actually normal and healthy. It's using food too often to get that time-out that becomes problematic.

Later in this book, when you go through the sessions, we'll explore other, nonfood ways for you to get the time-out you need to calm down, think clearly about your situation, and choose a powerful action.

SHRINK YOURSELF SESSION NOTES

The Feeling Phobia and Food Trance

- You've begun to identify your feeling phobia.
- You've started to think about what you make your feelings mean, your misinterpretations, your catastrophe predictions, and your powerlessness conclusions.

- You've identified the benefits of being in the food trance: the escape it gives you and the pleasure it provides.

- You've examined what it costs you to retreat into the food trance instead of facing your feelings, especially the fact that it keeps you from solving the problems that need to be solved.

- You've begun to think about the possibility that there are other ways you can get a time-out when feelings become too intense.

- You have to remember that you need to master the feeling phobia and food trance in order to understand the deeper issues that make you feel powerless.

3

The Costs of
Powerlessness

Whatever is formed for long duration arrives
slowly to its maturity.—*Samuel Johnson*

Power versus Powerlessness

There are at least two different kinds of power for us to consider: the
power over others and the power over yourself. The first is your
power to influence or control events and circumstances outside
yourself. This power depends in large part on your role in life, and
the power invested in that role by the institution you work in. If
you're the president of the United States or Exxon or Goldman
Sachs, you have a lot of power to make changes within your own
institution and upon the larger world. But even in those exalted
power roles, the occupant can be powerless to make many of the
changes they would like to see happen. The point is that in every
role you have some power to influence the world, and some very
real limits to getting everything you want done the way you want it

and when you want it. That's life, and the same principles apply to the role of mother, father, boss, employee, laborer, or night watchman. That's the external world we live in and have to adapt to.

We can increase our powerfulness in the world in two ways. We can get ourselves promoted to a more powerful role, or we can become more skilled and competent in our role and thereby, by becoming more effective, become more influential.

The second kind of powerfulness is power over yourself, which means not just the obvious, to control and discipline yourself, but to let yourself be the author, the agent, the one in control of your own life. That's the powerfulness we'll be focusing on in this book as I show you how to maximize your power over yourself in order to end emotional eating and, as a side benefit, get a lot more out of your life. I can do this because I know how you're giving away your power over yourself unnecessarily, and covering over that fact by eating excessive amounts of food.

At those times when you give away your power over yourself, you experience one or more of the five different layers of powerlessness that we'll discuss in each of the five subsequent chapters.

You have a strong critical voice inside you that tells you in dozens of different ways that you don't have the complete set of rights to be in control of your own life, and when you believe that voice, you lose your courage. That's when you have the experience of powerlessness, and if you're an emotional eater, that's when the uncontrollable urge to eat occurs. That strong critical voice is really your conscience, which hasn't yet evolved enough to become the reliable useful guide to your self-authored life because you're still being measured by impossible perfectionist standards.

Bella is twenty-seven years old. She's 5'4" and weighs 140 pounds. She's the manager of a restaurant. She has her own apartment. She graduated in the top of her class at university. By most people's standards she's really successful, and yet every time she has to make a decision, anything from whether she should take a cab or the subway, to what kind of coffee table to buy, to whom she should date, she has to consult her friends. She doesn't believe she can make her own decisions. She doesn't feel like the author of her life in some areas even though she clearly has been in other areas. When she's faced with something that feels like a big decision and she can't get someone on the phone to coach her through it, she feels powerless and ends up eating. It's this sense of powerlessness in her ability to take charge of her own life that has had her take off and put back on twenty pounds time and time again. In order to make light of this painful pattern, she jokes with her friends that she's the human accordion.

Every time Bella listens to her critical conscience's impossible standards of perfection and fails to make a decision on her own, she confirms her innate fear that she is powerless.

Where Did the Voice That Makes You Powerless Come From?

In the beginning of your life you were truly powerless. When you were born, you had no sense of yourself as an individual. You didn't recognize yourself as separate from your parents—they were looming presences whom you could see, hear, touch, and make respond to you, but you experienced them as part of yourself. Also, because your parents produced you, according to the law, they virtually owned you. You were totally dependent on them for sustenance, protection, survival, and audience. When you discovered your own toes, your nose, your fingers, you experienced surprise and delight, but still had no concept of yourself as an individual being—you remained, essentially, an appendage of your parents.

All of your attention as a baby was directed toward your parents—watching them, learning from them, getting them to respond to your needs. You didn't judge their wisdom at that time—they represented God, the source of all knowledge and sustenance. Since your parents constituted your whole world, you figured out a way to "keep them with you" even when they left the room. You imagined them as if they lived inside you. You started mimicking them to keep them close. When you observe young children, you'll often hear them repeat to themselves what Mom or Dad said, in the parent's voice: "Great job." "I said no." "Don't drink in the living room."

And so, by the time you reached the ripe old age of two, you had internalized your parents. You knew what they thought about you, whether you were good or bad, and they spoke their opinions to you even when they weren't around, from your internalized image of them. You no longer needed your physical ears to hear Mom say, "Don't drink in the living room" when you made a mess; you told yourself "You're a bad boy," perhaps in Mom's voice, because Mom had become alive inside you.

You needed this internal critic in early life to keep you out of trouble. Mom told you not to touch the hot flame, and you internalized that instruction so that you didn't need her to stand over you every time you saw fire. Mom told you not to spit at people or stick your tongue out at them, that it's disrespectful to do that, and you internalized her scolding so that you didn't make enemies when you started kindergarten. If you hadn't obeyed your mother's warnings about the world in an absolute way, you couldn't have played outside later, you couldn't have walked to school when you got old enough, you couldn't have been trusted on your own. And so Mom and Dad's internalized rules helped you to navigate and survive in the new, sometimes dangerous and confusing universe you found yourself exploring.

All of the rules of life that you learned started out as rigid absolutes: all or nothing, black or white. These rules originated from outside you, but you internalized them and obeyed them even when others weren't watching. They became your values, your rules, your way of looking at life, and your conscience.

As long as you obeyed all the rules, you were rewarded with the illusion of absolute safety . . . somehow or other, powerful parents would protect you from all of the hazards of life. If you disobeyed, you would be abandoned, and would have to deal with all of the overwhelming dangers in your life all by yourself, without knowledge or borrowed resources. That was your emotional choice when you were two. Obey, and be magically protected. Disobey, and become powerless to survive. You can see the primitive origins of powerlessness in that scenario.

So that strong critical voice that is still telling you what you're allowed to do as an adult originally had absolute power over you early in your life because you didn't have the capacity to fend for yourself at age three. But as you grow up and become more competent to lead your life your way, you can fend for yourself, and flourish. It's your conscience that still lags behind, and has to be updated to match your age and competency. But that's not easy to do.

Helping Your Conscience Grow

Under normal, healthy circumstances, you wouldn't have continued honoring those same rigid rules forever. They would have become modified by experience, contextualized. Most rules that made sense for you as a two-year-old no longer apply when you turn twelve. By then you have the competency and the right to walk across the street by yourself, for instance, even when there's no stoplight. You have real, albeit limited, power to take charge of certain parts of your life, like walking to school.

By the time you reach age twenty or thirty, the rules have been changing daily as new experiences require you to adapt to a world you couldn't imagine a decade before. You can swear freely when the time calls for it; you can choose to ignore Aunt Isabel because she constantly criticizes you; you can elect to leave your clothes piled on the chair until tomorrow. As an adult, you have the option to make your own rules after questioning and modifying and learning the hard way by making mistakes and being awkward.

And so, you would expect that you'd simply disregard the old rules and implement new, adult ones, except that every single time you modify some internalized rule, every time you change a rule to make it your own or drop a rule that doesn't make sense to you, you face an anxiety challenge. For instance, think about what you experienced in owning your adult sexuality. As a child, you couldn't touch anyone sexually, maybe even yourself, without evoking a rebuke. As a teen, you got bombarded with straight talk, warnings, and prohibitions about sex. By the time you became old enough to engage in adult sexual activity, you needed to rewrite the script and give yourself permission to go ahead in spite of the internalized voice telling you that sex leads to some version of hell. For many people, making that leap means overcoming considerable anxiety.

When you convert an old rule into your own value, you take authority away from your internalized owner and transfer it to yourself, the new owner. This is how you become your own person—by undergoing this step-by-step process in which you become the owner of your own rules. In so doing, you diminish the original authority that actually represents a version of your internalized parents. So anytime you create your own rules and challenge the rigid strictures that you've been living by, in a sense you're standing up to your parents and daring to be on your own. This means that you give your internalized parents a pink slip, and that can cause palpitations for even the most healthy among us. You're sacrificing the illusion of safety in order to be free to live your own life.

The job of the critical conscience is to keep you as safe as a rule-abiding child. The critical conscience wants to remain intact as an extension of your parents' mind-set, values, and historical view of life—a replica of what they contend you need to be in order to be loved and to not be abandoned. Meanwhile, your job is to assert your individuality and freedom by deciding what is right or wrong, good or bad, useful or not useful, based on your evolving view of life during your journey through the life cycle. You can see that you and your critical conscience have competing agendas.

There's a natural tension between your need to evolve and your own critical conscience's need to keep you from striking out on your own. Your critical conscience tries to scare you into not taking risks or venturing out on your own. Yet you have a defiant need for freedom that fuels you into rebellion. It's as if you have two powerful creatures dueling it out in your body, in your mind.

In the last chapter we talked about how people make their feelings, circumstances, and interactions with people mean something. They don't generally interpret things in their favor, though; in fact, they often interpret things in a way that confirms their worst fears, which is why we call it a misinterpretation. The way that you'll begin to mature the critical conscience is by understanding that there are two things that happen when you feel something, or when something happens in your life. There is your internal reality, the ways in which you measure what you're feeling or what has happened against everything else that has ever happened in your life, who you think you are, and who you'd like to be. Then there is the external reality, which is what is actually happening. To really look at what's actually happening, you need to weigh all sides of a feeling or situation. Take Bella, who we mentioned earlier in this chapter. When she's faced with a decision that feels difficult to make and she can't get a friend on the phone to consult with, she can immediately turn toward food because she feels too powerless to make any kind of decision on her own, or she can weigh all sides of what's actually happening. She can understand that her friends are busy. She can write a pro-and-con list and try to make a decision on her own. If possible, she can delay making her decision. I call this process of looking at all sides of something before immediately assuming you're powerless a "reinterpretation." It's not falsely interpreting something simply to put things in your favor; it's interpreting something from a real-life point of view, assuming that our initial interpretation of anything is generally based more on our internal reality, and so much of that is rooted in the past.

To interrupt the immediate need to eat, you'll learn to slow down long enough to look at what's going on in your inner reality and what's going on in the external reality, and then reinterpret things in such a way that you'll be able to own your power and become the author and agent of your life.

Once Bella was able to start making reinterpretations, she no longer felt that she needed someone every time there was a decision to be made. Sure, she still likes weighing all sides of things with her friends, but she has learned to trust her own ability to make choices and decisions for herself.

Freedom to Be Yourself

If all goes well, your critical conscience loses. You evolve and grow, the end point being that you have no more harsh, unrealistic, perfectionistic, absolute rules to live by or criteria to meet—just a good set of values and guidelines and rules of thumb to help you decide what to do and how to behave. You develop a friendly, mature conscience based not on fear and outdated notions, but instead on your experience in the world. Your conscience nudges you a bit when you slip, reminds you to give to the poor, to help someone even when it isn't convenient, and to avoid certain temptations because they're too risky or potentially hurtful to those you love. The ideal end point is 100 percent self-ownership so that you can deal with reality straight on, with an open creative mind, not hampered by outdated, rigid ways of looking at the world. In other words, your naturally evolving self puts your critical conscience out of business and replaces it with you, who, in an ideal world, handles challenges in a straightforward, adult manner, without resorting to food addiction. But, alas . . .

If you've been using food to shut down rather than transcend your critical conscience (because you don't want to hear its perfectionistic self-accusations about your worth, your adultness, your style, your friends, your anger, your lovableness, your values, or your impulses or its pessimistic projections about your dreams, your ambition, and your ability to handle life), you've stopped or seriously slowed down the natural and necessary separation from your critical conscience. You may have quieted the strong critical voice when it acts up too vigorously by eating, but you remain stuck with its criticisms and demands as soon as the food gets digested.

In the next chapter, I'll help you see how you can move the dial forward in your quest for independence by addressing the self-doubts that your critical conscience relies on to control you. Think of it this way: there are three stages in the development of your conscience. You've mastered the first—you no longer obey every single rule your parents taught you, so your conscience is not the absolute master of you as it was when you were three. You are in the long second stage, where you and your nagging critical conscience are in contention for control. You are heading for the third stage, where the nagging and false accusations are a thing of the past, and your conscience represents your values and integrity. So from now on, every time we refer to your conscience, we are talking to you about this second stage.

SHRINK YOURSELF SESSION NOTES
Unnecessary Powerlessness

- You've begun to see that it's you who makes you feel powerless.
- The part of you that measures yourself by impossible standards, making you temporarily powerless, is an overly harsh conscience.
- You've started to realize that if you eat to avoid self-accusations rather than confront them, you never get a chance to reform and remodel your conscience.

4

Your Self-Doubt Layer

No one can make you feel inferior without your consent.
—*Eleanor Roosevelt*

My patient Carmen was out shopping with her single friend Lucy after Carmen's son was born. They were both excited because the famous European clothes store H&M had just opened in New York. Lucy picked out her size 4 clothes, and Carmen picked out her barely fitting size 14s. As they were trying things on in the dressing room side by side, Lucy glanced sideways at her friend and said, "Carmen, perhaps you'd have better luck at a store for umm, bigger women, like Lane Bryant or The Avenue." Carmen felt angry at Lucy, but actually it wasn't Lucy's offense per se that made her feel terrible. If Carmen weren't already feeling so uncomfortable with her postbaby body, if her weight hadn't been such an issue since she was a child, if she hadn't had a history of comparing herself to Lucy since they were cheerleaders together in high school, then Lucy's comment might not have hurt so much, and she might not have needed to immediately grab an ice cream cone the minute she left the store.

Let's say someone breaks a date with you. You probably start a self-critical judgment that your mind finds too painful to deal with (He/she broke that date with me, what does he/she think is wrong with me?), so you run to food for refuge, then criticize yourself for overeating and end up focusing on what you've just consumed rather than the message in the hurt feelings. That's why it's common to hear people complain about how angry they are at themselves for having gone on a binge. It's easier to live with a self you've deemed temporarily lacking in self-control than with a permanently stupid or ugly self that nobody wants to spend time with. In psychoanalytic language, this is called a displacement—a little trick of the mind to reduce the interior pain level connected to self-doubt.

A little displacement is all right temporarily, but when it comes to food addiction there is no such thing as a little displacement. It doesn't work because you actually bury the self-doubt under food and make it almost unavailable to your conscious mind. You're unable to grapple with the self-accusation that you're a defective human being (ugly, or stupid, or unlovable, as you might be if someone broke a date with you). Unless you confront these overly harsh self-assessments (that part of your conscience that's still operating at a critical level), you actually believe them, and soon you stand accused and convicted without the benefit of an open trial. Who wouldn't want to suppress such a verdict with food and then more food? Who wouldn't rather think that they're just a person with no willpower than a person that is completely unworthy of love? It's normal to choose the former. But it's wrong.

You Measure Yourself from the Inside Out

As human beings, we like to measure things. Anyone who has a child knows that a broken cookie is just not the same thing as a whole cookie. It doesn't give the same sense of satisfaction—it actually doesn't taste the same. Ask children to pick a piece of dessert off a plate or a toy out of a bag and they'll ask for the biggest one. As we get older, we continue to measure not just the size of things, but also the quality, the appearance, the monetary value of everything, including ourselves. And as we judge, so we are judged.

You've been measured and judged ever since you were a child. Were you a good enough student for your parents or teachers? Were you pretty enough or handsome enough, kind enough, loving enough, a good enough athlete? Naturally, you came up short in some categories—we all do. The unfortunate thing is that inevitably you learned to judge yourself as others judged you. If you're like most people, you can hardly get through a day without making some negative assessment of yourself. You see a younger or more attractive or smarter person and you compare yourself, and at least momentarily you think you aren't good enough. You don't measure up. And when you measure, you probably don't measure fairly—you compare one of your weak areas against one of someone else's strongest areas.

Your opinions of yourself as a child were so dependent on what your parents, teachers, and friends thought of you, but as you get older, you have to develop a solid sense of who you are separate from the opinions of others. Of course, that doesn't mean you'll be immune from what others say or do, but it'll make you less susceptible to feeling awful and having a feeding frenzy when someone says they don't like what you're wearing.

If you're an emotional eater, every time you determine you aren't good enough, you become hungry. Feeling inadequate is as powerful a hunger stimulant (phantom hunger) as low blood sugar or a day without eating (biological hunger). Of course, there are other emotional factors that can stimulate your desire for food that we've yet to explore, but insecurity outranks other issues by a long shot, and it has a tricky way of masquerading as other things.

For instance, you may think you crave almond croissants because your husband tears you down verbally and you want a sweet comfort, but actually, you eat the croissants because you believe the ridiculous things he says about you. It's your own lack of self-esteem that triggers the eating. It's not what he says. If your sense of self were more valuable than his opinion of you, you'd ignore him, and the croissants as well.

Or suppose you find yourself bored and wanting something to eat instead of trying something new or interesting. You may lack confidence to even explore a new idea. Or if you eat out of anger, say because your neighbor's dog won't stop barking, you eat because you fear the outcome of a confrontation, something that could reflect badly on you. It throws you into a state of self-doubt. If your anger arises when your wife asks you to stop driving so fast, the real, underlying trigger might be that you feel uncertain about something else, so even a simple criticism becomes too much of an assault on a sore and sensitive ego.

As you further delve into all of this you may discover that the single biggest problem standing between you and a thin body has to do with your harsh view of yourself. This may seem to be a strange focus for a book about weight, but the measurement of your interior self has a lot more to do with the measurement of your waist than you might realize. The emotions that your mind transforms into phantom hunger all connect to your interior life, with self-doubt as the central organizer. If food has become your major mood-regulating mechanism, you'll find yourself overeating every time your mood slips, every time you feel you don't measure up, every time you think you or your life aren't good enough.

Self-Doubts Triggered by Others

Someone's opinion of you does not have to become your reality.
—*Les Brown*

I have a patient who traveled in Thailand for a year, only having brief interactions with other travelers. Her weight was never an issue while she was away and she came back weighing her ideal weight, almost effortlessly. When she returned she said, "It's amazing. Nothing bothered me while I was there and so I didn't struggle with food at all. My mother wasn't calling me telling me all the things that are wrong with my life. I wasn't in a love relationship. There was no one to criticize my job performance. I was so focused on meeting new people, meditating, and seeing things that I only ate when I was actually hungry."

This is not a suggestion that you should leave your family and friends and live in isolation if you want to lose weight. Anyone can be a Buddha on a mountaintop with no one or nothing around to trigger them. It's the person who can be a Buddha at their mother-in-law's kitchen table who is more likely to reach enlightenment.

Nothing activates self-doubt like getting criticized or rejected by other people, and so that's where we'll start. Even confident people slip onto shaky ground when they feel rejected, and if you're an emotional eater, you'll quickly want a food fix after you get your feelings hurt. After Mom points out that you haven't been on a date in twenty-seven months, you may go home and eat three brownies. You might feel angry at your mother and blame her for making you feel terrible, but experience has shown me that it isn't an insult or offense *per se* that triggers emotional hunger. You could survive any insult slung in your direction if only you didn't allow it to trigger your self-loathing. Who makes you feel miserable—your attackers? You can't really blame those who chastise or shun you for your brokenness; you can really only blame yourself. You're the one who makes yourself feel worthless. Let me explain.

When you experience rejection or criticism, first you suffer pain from the hurtful incident, and that triggers the old tape loop inside your head that tells you that you really are a loser, and that's why people treat you so poorly. You jump right onto the rejection band-wagon and believe the worst about yourself, rather than the best, and you can't bear feeling that way. Even if you don't buy the critical message you receive—if you don't agree with Mom that you should be married because "at age thirty you ain't no great catch anymore"—you allow her negative message to trigger other negative beliefs you have about yourself. Maybe Mom's criticism makes you worry that nobody will ever love you or that you'll never truly love anyone (catastrophe predictions), or that there's something wrong with you for not wanting to be married, or that something's wrong with you for getting so angry at your mom, or even for having such a terrible mom in the first place. When it comes to finding ways to reject ourselves, we're a remarkably creative species.

Hurting Yourself because Someone Else Hurt You

You need to separate the experience of *being hurt* from the experience of *hurting yourself in response to being hurt,* so you can see the difference. It's the judgment you make about yourself that hurts so much, and that is what drives you to eat. It's painful self-doubt that grumbles in your phantom stomach. Disappointments and rejections are real-world phenomena that can be handled in many different ways. But self-doubt is something else. It's harder to nail down; it's deeply entrenched and very painful. It's the thing we're so afraid of. It triggers our feelings of powerlessness because if we're really as awful as we think and we have no power to change, then life is simply too overwhelming to bear. We need an escape, any one we can find, and food is generally the most accessible option.

Each of us has particular vulnerabilities that trigger our worst thoughts about ourselves. You might fall apart when your husband forgets to kiss you good night, taking it as confirmation that you're completely undesirable. Your friend might go nuts when her boss refuses her promotion request, interpreting that to mean that she has no talent. The trick is to know what makes you "crazy insecure." If you know what triggers you, you can intervene before you react by overeating.

Let's say you get home from work after a difficult day and your spouse criticizes you or acts cold and distant. At the office, you handled one annoying phone call after another, then your boss asked you to redo the project plan that you had worked on all month, and on your way home, you got stuck in traffic for forty-seven minutes with a broken radio. You want a little comfort and support, but instead your spouse has the television on and barely looks up when you walk in the door. No kiss, no "Welcome home," no hot meal waiting. Your spouse's behavior leaves you hurt, disappointed, and at least a little bit angry. So you go to the kitchen, eat a piece of cheese, last night's chicken, four cookies, the kids' leftover pizza, and six bites of ice cream. For a few minutes you forget about your day, your boss, the traffic, your lazy husband, and your annoying kids, but then there's this nagging voice inside that reminds you that you just blew your diet and that by opting for the eating solution, you have also avoided finding some better solution to your disappointment. Now you can deal with all of your bad feelings by putting the television on and zoning out, or you can go to bed, or you can eat more. All of those solutions numb your feelings for the moment, but none of them solve anything; your bad mood is likely to get carried into the next day.

What would happen if, instead of eating, you could freeze-frame your feelings and put them under the microscope at the moment the tension occurs? Like the woman above who came home from a stressful day of work, most likely you'd see that you initially feared that your partner had some valid reason for ignoring you—you feared that your partner was cold because there was something unlovable (self-doubt label) about you and so you deserved the rejection. If you were able to slow down instead of immediately using food to ease the blow, you might be able to make a reinterpretation.

You might see that perhaps your husband had a hard day at work, too. Perhaps he could sense your angry mood and was afraid that anything he said would be wrong. From that thoughtful place, where you don't immediately get disappointed or make an assumption that what's happening is about you, you might be able to ask your husband for a hug or call a friend to talk about your day, something that would actually help you feel better rather than just distracting you. It's human to doubt yourself; we all have places where our confidence wavers, although during normal day-to-day life we usually keep our self-doubts under control, at least to a degree, so that we can function. But rejection or criticism or disappointment startle the self-doubts awake, and they really hurt when they're activated. As soon as you experience hurt feelings and accompanying self-doubt, you grab food to appease yourself. In fact, your pain may so quickly get transformed into hunger that you don't even recognize the pain that initially triggered the hunger. We will work toward slowing down and reinterpreting what has happened so that you don't hurt yourself in the same way that you've just been hurt by someone.

Unprovoked Self-Doubts

I have an inferiority complex, but it isn't a very good one.—Anonymous

Sometimes, even when there's no one around to provoke you, you might still feel horrible about yourself. In fact, for some of you, you may feel more horrible when you're alone. Self-doubt needs no other person, no slight or rejection, in order to make an appearance.

Judy, the forty-three-year-old mother of three, says that after all her kids go to sleep she feels so unfulfilled, and then she feels guilty and that makes her feel like a bad mother. She finds herself sitting on the couch when the house is quiet eating M&Ms and watching reality television.

You can have a self-doubt dream in the middle of the night and wake up craving food. You can sit alone in the park and obsess about what's wrong with you, convicting yourself for being a bad parent or spouse or friend. You can become paralyzed by critical words you hear inside your own head—words spoken to you decades ago by critics long dead. It's as if an inner detractor resides inside you, taking up where the critical parent or teacher left off. You hear the verdict leveled against you, but not the deliberations, and so you give yourself no chance to put forth a defense. Self-doubts can be so overwhelming that nothing seems to help: even if others contradict your doubt, you can't take it in.

Camille, a thirty-one-year-old social worker, has spent her whole life helping people. In high school everyone called her to talk about their problems; she supported her college boyfriend through medical school and was then surprised when he left her for a co-worker at the hospital; she even made a career out of putting her needs aside by becoming a social worker. Camille believes that unless she's helping people, they won't want to be around her. Being the helper is Camille's armor. It covers up for the fact that she doesn't think she's worthy of having anyone do anything for her.

In order to deal with the pain of feeling inadequate and unworthy, many of us develop a type of defense that I call "the armor." Your armor is a role or persona you adopt in order to shield yourself from the pain of self-doubt. However, armor represents a false front, and often it's a dysfunctional front. It also prevents us from really feeling fulfilled in relationships because even if someone loves our armor, we secretly know that they wouldn't love the person who is hiding underneath. For instance, you might adopt a victim role in order to shield yourself from your self-doubts, unconsciously feeling that if people realize how pathetic and needy you are, they'll lay off you. Obviously, you can't challenge anyone from your victim position—you can't grow or change—and so in the end, your armor gives you one more thing to feel bad about, one more thing to instigate an eating binge. Likewise, if you adopt a workaholic armor with the unconscious motivation of being too exhausted to face your self-doubts because every waking moment is spent compensating for and proving them wrong, then you'll end up spiritually bereft and emotionally hungry.

Some of the common types of armor that people wear are the following: martyr, nurturer, perfectionist, loner, clown. Wearing the armor can become so habitual that you mistake the alias for your true self. It's useful to identify the type of armor you wear, so that you can begin stepping out of it to address the self-doubt head-on. Until you allow your true self to emerge, you won't feel loved and you won't believe in the love that people are offering.

Meet Harriet, Your Self-Critic

Let's call the self-critical voice inside you "Harriet" or "Harry." You can rename this inner censor anything you want, but for the sake of simplicity, let's just call her Harriet for now. Of course, you don't really have a person named Harriet living inside your bones, but you do have an inner critical voice that might as well be another person, because like a person, this inner critic has a certain consistency in its attitudes and judgments and it functions as an entity within you, influencing your actions and beliefs about yourself. Take a moment now to imagine that the self-critical voice in your head has a personality and even the name Harriet. Try to listen to the self-deprecating messages that Harriet is giving to you even at this very moment. She rarely rests.

Even though you're an intelligent, self-contained, functioning adult, Harriet has a lot of power. Sometimes her chatter stays in the background of your consciousness, like static, but other times it's blaring like a sports announcer, really berating you. You need to get her under control in order to control your emotional eating pattern. As a psychiatrist, when a patient is coming in every week talking about their self-doubts, directly or indirectly, I make it a point to maintain the perspective that they're a person who despite their doubts also has successes in their life: they have a job, a spouse, a family, hobbies, interests, passions. So I'm going to ask you to treat your inner critic Harriet by being sure to have a dialogue with her that's surrounded by this same reality perspective. No matter what she says, you must always go back to your reality. It's your anchor in the world of today that will keep you sane and strong. Like a good therapist, you have to remember all your good qualities and victories. From that perspective, you'll be in a much better place to hear what Harriet has to say and think about what it means, rather than run for the hills every time she opens her mouth.

My working assumption is that you know Harriet quite well but have never figured out how to handle her, other than trying to avoid doing anything to stimulate one of her verdicts. You've become accustomed to living with her inside you, and when she's become too intense or aggressive, you've tried to shut her up by eating or drinking your way into oblivion. You've used food to try to stuff Harriet down and maybe even alcohol to poison her. These substances allow you to go into a sort of trance where you can't hear Harriet's voice anymore.

You've been suffocating and poisoning Harriet because she seems dangerous to you—because until now, you've granted her the status of a goddess. Whatever she's said, you've believed without question. If Harriet has whispered that you're inept or a loser or not likeable, you've accepted those judgments. You go ahead and eat another piece of cake because Harriet has convinced you that whatever diet you're on is never going to make a real difference. She's convinced you that you'll never lose the weight and that even if you do lose the weight, people still won't love you the way you want them to. You haven't been able to talk back to Harriet any more than you could talk to an enraged parent making the same pronouncements about you—you wouldn't dare. You've assimilated Harriet's harsh and unfair criticisms as basic truths about yourself, the proof of your badness and your defectiveness. But now you've given Harriet an ordinary mortal name and taken her down a notch, so you can begin exploring whether or not she's telling the truth.

In fact, Harriet is your conscience, or in psychological terms, what we call the "superego." This is not your whole conscience, but that sector that still operates on an immature level. She's a part of you, not a concrete thing exterior to you or a mysterious, powerful "other" inside you. You're telling yourself something highly critical about yourself, and you believe it without question. You assume your conscience is infallible, elevated, and even godlike, but while your mature conscience helps you to behave with decency in the world, the critical conscience, Harriet, always goes overboard in assigning guilt.

How to Weaken the Power of Your Self-Doubts

There are two ways to weaken the power of your self-doubts. One is an interior conversation with yourself and Harriet, your inner critic, whenever you're in the midst of accusing yourself of something. We'll be giving you the scripts to dialogue with Harriet in Session 4 (chapter 13) of part two. This is one way that you'll be reinterpreting things and feelings in order to have a more accurate inner reality.

The other way to weaken your self-doubts is to stop automatically and mindlessly strengthening your self-doubts by jumping to conclusions that you don't examine as you interpret the world outside or yourself. When something happens—for instance, you're disappointed with yourself for doing a bad job at work and you jump to the conclusion that there's something wrong with you and then eat to avoid dealing with that conclusion—you reinforce your self-doubt. You're making an incorrect interpretation of the event just because you're disappointed in yourself, and because you've eaten to smother the feeling, you've robbed yourself of the opportunity to make a reinterpretation. You've compounded that self-doubt. The fact that you did a bad job at work doesn't mean that there's something wrong with you. It doesn't mean that you're lazy or stupid or incompetent—it simply means that you didn't do a good job at work. If you look at the exterior reality and weigh all the sides of what happened, you may realize that perhaps it means that you didn't put in enough effort to match the difficulty of the task, or you didn't have enough time to do it right, or you weren't really motivated to do it in the first place. Once you can see the real picture and make a reinterpretation, instead of just your knee-jerk immediate interpretation that leads you to the experience of powerlessness and then the uncontrollable urge to eat, you have some choices. You can apologize. You can commit to doing a better job the next time. You can realize that you're simply not motivated at your job and would rather be doing something else. When you do that, you regain your power. And regaining your power allows you to be your own agent in the world. How skilled you get at looking at the external world of today, rather than your interior world of your past where Harriet rules, will determine how much agency you actually have over your own life and ultimately over your weight.

In other words, imagine you're holding all your self-doubts and they're piled twelve layers high. Every time you dialogue with Harriet, you take a layer off with your right hand. Of course, I want you to take all the layers of your self-doubt away. But every time you immediately accept your misinterpretation of something, you're putting a layer back on with your left hand. The pile doesn't change and you're left with your self-doubts. By dialoguing with Harriet you'll take your existing self-doubts away, and every time you reinterpret something to reflect the real-life external reality of today, you'll be preventing a new layer from being put on.

Since your self-doubts are the first layer of the powerlessness experience that causes the uncontrollable urge to overeat, figuring out how to master your old self-doubts, not fear Harriet, and prevent new self-doubt from being added to your collection by embracing the external reality is the first key to success.

In part two, you'll actively attack Harriet by learning how to defend yourself against her accusations, but for now, it will help you to keep these three principles that we've discussed in mind:

1. Your self-doubts represent only a part of yourself, not the whole picture. Your self-doubts take your everyday mistakes and failures and inflate them so that they're unbearable. If you stay grounded in your real life, the self-doubt experience will be only a momentary experience without any effect, just a reflex that goes nowhere. My patient Roz is a published magazine writer. She got a critical note from her editor. Normally this would send her running to the fridge, her self-doubts from childhood about not being creative enough fully awakened. But after working with me, she was able to stop and realize that she's a good writer and that one criticism doesn't erase all her accomplishments. She went back to her desk, took her editor's comments to heart, and rewrote her piece. Her editor was pleased with it, and she didn't have to confront the guilt from overeating.

2. The second principle is that the self-doubt powerlessness experience lasts only as long as you continue to reinforce it by misinterpreting the daily events in your life. Every time you create a false link between the event (e.g., a rejection or disappointment and the conclusion there must be something wrong with you to explain why this is happening), you feed the self-doubt powerlessness conclusion. Every time you spend time thinking about and analyzing the situation to understand the real-life complex cause, you stay in the real world. The initial misinterpretation must be replaced with the correction reinterpretation. Roz

misinterpreted her editor's comment to mean she wasn't good enough; when she reinterpreted, she remembered that her editor generally loves her work and is actually on her side.

3. You actually have to listen to your harsh critic and learn a new way of talking back to it. In part two, I'll provide you with scripts you can practice, but for now, let's look at the six most common accusations that Harriet will make against you, so you can begin thinking about how you will have to respond to each.

Six Accusations You'll Learn How to Counter

1. If you're not perfect, you're deeply flawed.
2. You're trying to cover up and deny your real faults.
3. You're a phony.
4. You're a pretend adult and don't deserve the full rights of adulthood.
5. You know the good stuff about you isn't real.
6. Everybody knows what you're hiding.

SHRINK YOURSELF SESSION NOTES

Powerlessness and Self-Criticism

- You've seen that you have self-doubts. Some are triggered by others, some are unprovoked.

- You've begun to see that perhaps you're wearing armor to protect yourself from self-doubts.

- You've met your inner critic, Harriet, and understand that she's been keeping your self-doubts in place.

- You made a false conclusion when you decided that "you're powerless to do anything about your self-doubts." That false conclusion has made you hide or run away into food.

- You learned the six accusations Harriet makes against you.

- You understand that up until now you've accepted those accusations as truth, but now you know that you'll need to dialogue with those accusations to see if they're just old tapes replaying or if they actually pertain to who you are today.

- You understand that you have two methods of mastering your self-doubts:

  1. You can diminish what is there now by talking back to your nagging critical conscience.

  2. You can stop adding to your load of doubt by catching yourself when you misinterpret a situation to mean there is something wrong with you.

5

Your Frustration/Reward Layer

We human beings come into the world hardwired to seek passion and pleasure and fulfillment. From the moment of birth, we look for pleasure. We delight in the breast or bottle; we need touch to survive; we like soft blankets and toys; we love when people pay attention to us, entertain us, and make us laugh. Even as babies, we become passionate about things—about a parent or sibling; about a character on television like Elmo or Barney; about a particular blanket, pacifier, or toy. And as babies, we first experience the frustration of not always getting what we want when we want it. This frustration creates a certain degree of pain. Babies cry in response to pain, and usually get the frustration allayed fairly quickly—the bottle or breast arrives, the blanket or toy is found. As we get older, though, we're on our own in resolving frustration. Our needs increase, as do our desires, and it takes increasingly more work, diligence, and audacity to find the passion and pleasure and fulfillment we long for.

Until now, when you've felt frustrated with some part of your life, you've eaten to satisfy yourself because deep down you haven't thought you had the power to do anything to reverse the frustration, to get your real needs met, and to have the life you want. Perhaps this frustration has led you to chronic feelings of disappointment and anger, and over time those feelings have turned into depression. I want to help you see that you don't need to stay in this conundrum. You've come to the wrong conclusion. Although you'll always have frustrations in life, there's always something you can do to either diminish them, reverse them, or peacefully coexist with them. Eating to give yourself an illusory reward is always the worst possible way to deal with your frustrations, for as we have pointed out so many times already, your problems don't get better, new problems accumulate, more self-doubts get added to the pile and that makes you want to eat more, and then the whole added load of hating yourself for being fat comes into play.

Up until now, you've learned that you're afraid of where your feelings might take you, what they might lead you to realize about yourself and your life. You've seen how in the past you resorted to eating in order to avoid the discomfort of whatever you were feeling for a brief period. You ate to end a bad feeling such as sadness or fear. That bad feeling covered for a deep anxiety that you didn't want to face, usually some notion that you're a defective person, that your mythically exaggerated doubts about yourself represented the secret truth about you. If you follow that line of thinking, you can see that it extends to the idea that you are so defective that you'll never achieve satisfaction. And so when you have frustrated needs that don't get met, you eat instead of dealing with them, which ensures that they don't get met, plus you feel even more terrible about yourself.

You can see how this cycle plays out in the case of Susie, a patient of mine who struggled to lose weight for years. Anytime it was suggested that she eat less, she felt panicked. She couldn't imagine what else she might do that could provide her with the pleasure that food provided. And she was passionate about her food, too. The thought of what she would eat at the end of her workday actually kept her motivated throughout the day. The meal that awaited her was almost as enticing as the idea of meeting a lover.

The fact of the matter was that her needs had not been met for a long time in her marriage. She had no outlets that gave her a feeling of accomplishment. Despite many compliments about the clothes she designed and made for her children, she had not been brave enough to take them to local stores. In our work together, she began to look at ways to overcome her self-doubt so that she could ask for what she needed from her husband and begin getting her hand-made clothes out into the world. Once she took these steps and started deriving a sense of real satisfaction from her life, food moved from first to third on her list of sources of pleasure.

Like Susie, you also need to look at your self-doubts, put them aside, and see what your true needs and passions are. In part two, we'll work on what I will discuss here, which is your:

- unfulfilling relationships
- unfulfilled needs
- unlived potential
- stresses

Using Food to Deal with Unfulfilling Relationships

Romance like donut. Everybody hungry for donut. Everybody hungry for romance. But when romance over, you not feel so good, maybe vomit. Same with donut.—*Unknown*

Let me tell you about Cara, who couldn't find the love she so desperately wanted—a variation on the theme of having a relationship with its built-in frustrations.

At age forty-nine, Cara's love life looked bleak. She hadn't had a date in two years, and no prospects loomed on the horizon. She longed for an intimate partner, someone who could help out with the financial burden and house chores, someone she could snuggle with and talk to late at night. A while back she joined Match.com, but all the guys disappointed her except for one, Jack, with whom she did finally start a relationship. Jack had some good qualities—generosity; he was good to Theresa, Cara's sixteen-year-old; and he had nursed Cara back to health after her shoulder surgery. He was kind and all that, Cara thought, but he was in debt and far too needy. She had to end it because Jack got demanding about spending more time together, not understanding that Cara's job required that she work sixty, sometimes seventy or eighty hours a week.

No guys seemed to get that fact. Lately, Cara's work schedule had made it difficult for her to cook good meals at home or to exercise. She started eating out a lot, and the pounds found their way to her waistline. Her friends urged her to rejoin a dating service, but she pointed out that it hadn't worked before and so she saw no reason to bother now. She had her daughter to take care of, and her demanding work schedule, and so she'd just have to trust fate. Plus she wanted to hold off until she lost some weight before dating again. No guy would want to go out with someone forty pounds overweight, she told her friends over drinks. When her sister suggested that she should get some counseling, Cara exploded. She didn't need counseling, she told her sister—she needed some relief from all the pressure. After she hung up, she fixed herself a chocolate milkshake with whipped cream and stuck *You've Got Mail* in the DVD player. Halfway through the movie, she felt munchy, so she grabbed the bag of Mint Milanos and ate the entire thing.

When first in love, we feel full, our appetites fall away, and we want nothing other than the beloved. And yet, as the Irish folk song, "The Water Is Wide," reminds us, there's another part to the story: "But love grows old, and waxes cold, And fades away, like morning dew," go the words, and therein lies the problem. When love grows cold, we grow hungry, and it hardly takes a major frost in the relationship to activate emotional hunger. Once the radiance of new love fades, frustrations begin, and then emotional hunger has a field day.

Our deepest fears, frustrations, and disappointments come from our interactions with people, and especially from those people we love most. In chapter 4, we explored how to deal with the emotional hunger that gets triggered when other people hurt us, but relationships engender problems other than hurt feelings that lead us to overeat. Perhaps your partner simply doesn't communicate, and that frustrates you, or you don't get what you need from your partner on an ongoing basis. Perhaps your partner has behaviors that frighten or dismay or irritate you, or perhaps you're the one who botches things because you fear intimacy. Perhaps everything seems fine on the surface, but you find yourself wanting something more—maybe more romance, or more freedom, or more excitement. What can you do about the hunger related to these issues?

First you need to figure out if, in fact, relationship issues do underlie some of your eating behavior, because such frustrations can be subtle, and because you might have developed elaborate defenses to suppress such issues in order to maintain the status quo. Recognizing frustrations in relationships takes courage. We crave love and intimacy with all our being, and so we hate to admit it when things aren't completely fulfilling. We don't want to lose the love we do have, unless the lack of fulfillment has become so blatant that we have no choice. And so we hold onto imperfect partnerships, figuring that's the best we're going to do, meanwhile doing nothing much to make things better.

As the above story about Cara illustrates, many people reach for food when they think love is totally out of reach. Some unconsciously hope to fill the void inside themselves by eating delicious treats. Others actually make a conscious decision to eat rather than to relate. You've probably seen those bumper stickers that say, "Forget love. I want to fall in chocolate." People who think that way have decided that it's easier to get a hit of bliss from a cookie than to deal with the emotional demands of love. Food doesn't talk back, it never says no, it doesn't criticize you. I understand the temporary fix that food provides, and have seen my patients turn to it countless times, but food will never satisfy that basic human need to be part of an intimate, harmonious, and fulfilling relationship. Although food can give you a momentary feeling of fullness, it can't fill the void that wants to be filled with love and intimacy.

How Harriet, Your Inner Critic, Interferes in Your Relationships

Food has replaced sex in my life. Now I can't even get into my own pants!—Anonymous

You've Got Mail, The Notebook, Sleepless in Seattle, Must Love Dogs. What stands between you and such enduring cinematic love?

You probably know by now that Harriet the nag creates problems that keep you from enjoying lasting intimacy. As long as self-doubt tickles you, even if only in the innermost recesses of your awareness, all your relationships will be difficult. Self-doubt makes you overly sensitive to perceived slights because deep inside you feel damaged or unworthy. Self-doubt makes you withdraw too quickly, hide too much, become jealous and envious, give up too easily, and rationalize your actions. When insecure, you avoid reaching out, and you spend too much relationship energy protecting your self-image. You wear at least one suit of armor, a challenge to any partner. You want or need too much attention and acclaim, and you become angry and hurt when you don't get it. In short, you become exactly the type of partner you would never want to be with, and so it should come as no surprise when you end up alone or when your partner points out some of these faults.

I find that many of my patients run into trouble because they aren't ready to part with Harriet. They're still functioning from their critical, childlike conscience. They can't love themselves, much less another. They say that they know love takes work, but they don't really get what that means—that the bulk of the work needs to be inner-directed. At some level, they want a fairy tale, a perfect prince or princess to come along and make everything gorgeous, although they act the part of the wicked witch, driving suitors away or making the relationship more difficult. Until you wrangle with Harriet and feel truly worthy of love, until you believe in your own ability to be loving, and reliable, and a gem of a partner, until you know deep down inside that you're the kind of person you'd like to spend eternity with, relationship problems will hound you and you'll overeat to compensate.

Also, when you don't believe in your inherent worth, you'll fear exposure, which makes intimacy impossible. Getting close to another person means letting him or her see all of you, including your imperfections. If you don't love yourself, you'll fear that your partner will find out the so-called truth about you—that under the surface, you're really bad, that Harriet speaks the whole truth and nothing but the truth. You also fear that your partner will confirm Harriet's accusations—a prospect so terrifying that you consciously or unconsciously sabotage your own relationships.

I had a patient who decided she was going to use skydiving to overcome her fears. She thought that if she jumped enough times, she would no longer be afraid. After doing it many times, she realized she was supposed to be afraid of jumping out of a plane at 15,000 feet.

Relationships are no different. Any time you make yourself vulnerable, you can expect to be frightened. But any time you let fear overwhelm you or make you run away, you reinforce your negative self-image, convincing yourself that you're weak, fearful, and someone who can't succeed in love. The challenge is to face the fears and the self-doubt head-on.

Sometimes it's the armor you have put on to run away from Harriet that becomes the obstacle. Let me tell you about Brad.

Brad had a way with women. In fact, he had his way with so many women in the past five years that he had lost count. Last March, he had the hots for Marissa, but her husband, Stewart, got between them. Then he fell for Sandy, but her two children botched that relationship. He could deal with neither the kid factor nor with clingy women, which was what had ruined his infatuation with Alison. Why, he wondered, couldn't God just send him a beautiful, sexy, smart, compatible, independent, kid-free woman he could enjoy life with? He didn't want to get married or anything, but he was beginning to feel weird about his lack of long-term success with women. All of his friends were either married or living with some-one, and he had an uneasy feeling about being the only guy he knew who had never been with a woman for longer than 14 months, although he did love living the bachelor dream.

Recently, his friends George and Lynette had set him up with Delia, who seemed to be perfect in every way. She was attractive and funny and smart, and she shared his interests. But after a few months, she started asking him what he was thinking about all the time, trying to figure him out. Sometimes it almost seemed as if she could read his mind—it kind of spooked him how she knew so much about his feelings. He told her to back off, and she got sulky and then they fought. He didn't like a meddlesome woman—he just wanted to have fun, he said. Then she started in on what she called "his relationship issues."

"You're forty-one," she said to him, "and you can't sustain a relationship because you're scared out of your mind." That really got to him. He broke up with her that very night, and then she told him to grow up and said he didn't deserve her. She said she didn't want to be with someone dysfunctional.

That was a month ago and he hasn't asked anyone out since then. He tried not to think about Delia, but for some reason, their last fight kept bugging him. In fact, it bugged him so much that he didn't want to date at all, for fear of getting into a similar situation.

Brad's armor was his womanizing. It covered up his fear of intimacy, which arose from his extreme sensitivity. He feared the vulnerability of being known and watched. If he was known and watched he might be found out to be the fraud he was sure he was. As long as he stayed encased in his armor, without any dialogue with Harriet that might change his self-perceptions, he was bound to experience a series of endless disappointments, his emotional hunger would remain enormous, and he would overeat to reward himself for what he couldn't fix. If Brad doesn't confront his serial womanizing with therapy or real introspection, all of his doubts will keep being confirmed, and ultimately he will become a caricature.

The Common Denominator in All Your Relationships

Wake up to your own strength. Wake up to the role you play in your own destiny. Wake up to the power you have to choose what you think, do, and say.—Keith Ellis, Bootstraps

In any relationship that you want to improve, you have to start with the premise that you can only change yourself, and in so doing change the dynamic of the relationship. Only then is there a chance that your partner may change in exactly the way you want in response. Most people don't understand this, even though they have heard it a thousand times. Instead we ask, beg, demand that our partner change to please us. Simply put, it won't work.

My patient Pam, a midlevel manager in an advertising firm in Manhattan, has been married for three years and has begged her husband to not take it personally if she is in a rage when she gets home from work. She expected him to understand how stressful her work is and accept any way she treated him. That is an unrealistic kind of unconditional love to expect. When Pam realized that it was unfair of her to expect this from her husband and started controlling her anger in a mature way, her relationship changed dramatically. She ended up getting many more of her needs met and was actually able to enjoy her time in the evenings after she came home from work. They even started taking walks every night after dinner, which has helped her relax even more and she's lost weight effortlessly.

Harriet stands in the way of you making changes. If Harriet were not in the picture, you could change your own behavior in your frustrating relationship and reap the rewards. You would

- try to open an honest dialogue
- expect less from your partner
- accept that you have different opinions on certain topics
- learn to not take things so seriously
- call your partner more often

- not be so stubborn or hard-headed
- not try to control everything
- let your partner have more space
- acknowledge that he or she is temporarily under a lot of stress

Instead of doing these things, we have such unrealistic expectations in love. Why do we want to be swept off our feet without putting forth any effort? We took the fairy tales that we heard when we were young to heart. We grew up expecting blissful, perfect, soul-matey love, and now, when our partners act like mere, imperfect mortals, we think the sky is falling. We feel angry, slighted, and, deep inside, inadequate—because we think we must be ugly frogs down to our bones or else we would have fairy-tale partners who treat us like royalty.

One way you can improve relationships and diminish emotional hunger is to get real about your relationships, including about your expectations of others. First you have to accept your own faults and realize that they don't add up to the entire you, and then you have to accept that your partner has faults that most likely comprise only part of the picture of who he or she is.

Going back to Pam, whom I mentioned above, it was her own change of attitude that got her relationship to improve so dramatically. A relationship with a difficult partner can change completely if you make minor adjustments in your attitude and behavior. There are two ways to do this:

One, if frustrated with a relationship, there are things you can do, and they all involve some change in you, your attitude, your behavior, your sensitivity, or your intimacy skills. You need to work on these instead of eating. You don't have to solve them all at once, though. Making small changes can actually offer a lot of relief, and you may not feel the need to immediately turn to food for that relief.

Second, you have to stop Harriet if she tries to prevent you from making these changes. You have to do combat with her or you won't be able to change, and your original conclusion that your frustrations can't be resolved will become correct. If that occurs, you'll be stuck and then you'll only continue eating to reward yourself for your frustrations.

Talk Back to Harriet

As you discover ways to improve your relationships, here are some of the things that Harriet may say about the things you are thinking of trying. I'd like to share them with you so that when Harriet starts suggesting them, you'll already be prepared with responses.

First, when you think that having a dialogue with a loved one is going to help, Harriet will warn you to be careful. She'll tell you that you might hear something about yourself that you can't quite handle. What will you tell her?

When you attempt to give your loved ones space, she'll tell you that if you don't have a hold over them they'll find someone else, or that by giving them space they'll find others more interesting and will eventually abandon you.

When you entertain the idea that perhaps you've been expecting too much from your loved ones, she'll tell you that by expecting less from people, you'll allow yourself to become a doormat. You'll be used because they know you're not worth anything more.

When you try to accept that people in your life are going to have different opinions, she'll tell you that if you have opposing opinions you'll be cast aside. Your opinions don't count after all.

When you try to lighten up and not take things so seriously, Harriet will tell you that if you don't take your feelings seriously, people will not pay attention to them. She'll encourage you to stay in an angry place where you feel lonely and disconnected.

When you try to stop being so stubborn and hard-headed, Harriet will tell you that you are compromising and that by giving in you are accepting that you're flawed and imperfect. Obviously, imperfect is bad by her standards.

When you give up trying to control everything and everyone (your spouse, your children, your co-workers), Harriet will tell you that if you relinquish control, things will go wrong and you'll look bad.

When you try to be sympathetic toward someone in your life who is under stress, Harriet will start to pout, saying, "What about me, where is my unconditional love and support?" When you're starting to feel bad about not receiving that kind of support, she'll convince you that you don't have it because you don't deserve it.

Harriet works hard to convince you that nothing is going to help in your relationships. She keeps you locked in a rigid pattern that never has things change or get better. To break free of her negative influence, spend some time planning counterarguments for any of her attacks. Ultimately, having good relationships is the highlight of life, the source of deepest fullness and fulfillment.

"Hormones," says Claire, a forty-two-year-old patient, when I ask her why she feels depressed.

"Is there anything else," I ask, "anything specific bothering you?"

Claire thinks for a moment. "I feel like something is wrong, but I'm not sure what it is."

My patient Richard comes in angry, cranky. "What's wrong?" I ask him.

"Nothing," he says. "I'm just in a rotten mood."

"What's causing the mood?"

"I don't know," says Richard. "That's why I'm paying you, to figure it out."

On a daily basis, patients like Richard and Claire tell me that they feel irritable and grouchy, but even when pressed, they really don't know what's making them miserable. They describe a free-floating feeling of discomfort that eats at them and makes them want to eat, but have no complaints grand enough to account for their misery. And so we do the work of exploring, digging for answers, and reflecting. Finally, we discover unfulfilled needs and desires buried deep beneath the surface. Those desires and needs, when not addressed, cause depression, anger, frustration, and, of course, hunger—a desire to fill the gap with food.

One of our online members wrote, "I wanted food to be so much more than nourishment. Food became the soother, the lover, the caregiver, gave me something to do when I was bored and didn't want to examine the direction of my life. Of course food isn't any of these things, 'it is just food.' I stuffed myself to fill all the gaps in my life rather than dealing with the gaps themselves. It wasn't until I realized that food wasn't any of those things that I was making it, it was just food, that I lost quite a bit of weight."

Most of us hunger for something that we lack. Maybe you want more security, or more appreciation, or more leisure in your life—but there's a good chance that you don't fully acknowledge or even know what you want. My experience working with patients over three decades has shown me that if you don't know what you want and if you fail to consciously own your desires, you'll find emotional hunger attacking you with ferocious strength.

In this frustration/reward cycle, we're following the consequences of the powerlessness conclusion that you cannot do anything about your frustration except to reward yourself with food. Well, when you feel frustrated but don't know why, it's true that you can't do anything about it. Perhaps you're even afraid to look for an answer because you fear that looking will lead you to an unbearable destination, to a place where you find out what you need but believe you'll never get it. No matter how scary that is, the cure is to dig and find out which of your needs are being frustrated, put those needs into words, and then figure out what to do about them.

You will have to determine which of your needs are infantile and unrealistic and which ones you should pursue getting met. The process of excavating and facing them is all you need to begin to stop the phantom hunger created by frustrated needs.

Remember, all of your legitimate needs cry out to be satisfied. When you frustrate a real need, you'll experience emotional hunger. You can create the temporary illusion that everything is all right for a while by eating, but food alone won't fulfill any need but physical hunger.

Your Needs Need to Mature, Too

Life is a process of becoming, a combination of states we have to go through. Where people fail is that they wish to elect a state and remain in it. This is a kind of death.—*Anaïs Nin*

One reason that you may lose touch with your needs or become frustrated that they'll never be satisfied is that you haven't changed your needs to adapt to the way your life has changed. For example, as a child, you were quite dependent on the approval of your parents. You constantly waited to hear your parents say "great job" after everything you did—everything from going down a slide, to coloring a picture, to making poopie in the potty—and you needed that validation.

As you got older, you undoubtedly received less validation. Adults simply can't expect to receive as much validation as kids get. Validation must become internal. You need to cheer for yourself. Your boss won't tell you "great job" every time you write a memo, your spouse won't exclaim with praise every time you smile—you have to enjoy yourself for your own accomplishments. Still, it's normal to need some external validation. If you gave your spouse an amazing fortieth birthday party and you got no acknowledgment, your need for thanks is an adult need that must find a way to be satisfied. Being able to look at your needs in a realistic and fair way is essential to your happiness and to the success of your relationships.

It's quite natural for your needs and dreams to shift to reflect your new life circumstances, and also typical to ignore this fact and keep acting as if the old needs apply. Every time you enter a transitional stage in your life, it's time to reassess and recalibrate your path—to assess what your needs have become and to look at which needs no longer apply.

What you might really need now is an opportunity to exercise your strength and independence. You may need a stage to play on now rather than a hiding place. And so it's important to assess whether your needs and desires are outdated—if they're tied to childhood fears rather than rooted in present reality.

Lois, a thirty-eight-year-old online member, doesn't struggle with her weight, but she does struggle with her relationship to food. She thinks about food constantly and binges occasionally, and then feels horrible guilt and shame for days. Even though she manages a business from her home and is the star tennis player at her club, she turns into a little girl around her husband. She expects him to handle the bills, take care of the cars, and even pitch in with her work whenever she feels overwhelmed. It's almost as if she forgets how competent she actually is when she's around him. Whenever he's not around and she has to do things for herself, she ends up bingeing.

If you identify with this, you'll need to stop looking for a protector and start looking for a stage. The change in your personal needs at any point in time is related to your place on the life stage spectrum. At each stage in the life journey, certain needs typically become relevant, although they weren't before. In your late teens, you are busy experimenting with adulthood and need both independence and family support in your half-child, half-adult status. In your twenties, the task is to become independent by becoming more competent at work and in love and friendships, and what you need is opportunity, experience, and hands-off acceptance of your method of learning about life. In your early thirties you need commitment and an opportunity to go deeper into your life and into yourself, often involving children and family life. In midlife, you might experience the need for professional success and fulfillment—many people do at this point in their life journey—whereas later life typically brings an increased longing for downtime and inner reflection.

One patient said, "Once my son left home, I didn't know how to fill my time. I felt lost, bored, and didn't know what I needed to make myself happy, and most times I just ended up eating to fill the time." Constantly reassessing your needs is part of what it takes to keep evolving and growing as an adult.

The key is to get in touch with your real needs at each point in your journey, and to recognize the legitimacy of your current needs so you can move forward. Although you might discover that you can't fulfill all your desires at this moment given the circumstances of your life, you at least can begin to construct a plan that works for you in your current situation.

Knowing What You Want So You Can Go for It

You might be saying I would go after what I need and want if only I knew what I needed or wanted. The real trouble begins when you no longer know what you want—when you lose touch with your dreams because they seem so impractical. This is a very common problem. We get too busy to take time for ourselves—we become caught up in life. We go through the motions of existence, spinning wildly on the hamster wheel of obligations and daily tasks, forgetting what we started out hoping for, burying ourselves in routine and work.

One of my patients recently said, "I take care of my three children with the grace of Mary Poppins. I make sure they explore all their interests. Why, then, can't I do that for myself?"

We may forget that we had any dreams at all. Then our old friend Harriet the naysayer reinforces our amnesia by making us feel that we aren't deserving and therefore should just accept life as it is. Meanwhile, the dreams we once had nag at us, or new needs bubble up, and though we ignore them, we feel frustrated, which breeds depression and anger.

Dig beneath the surface of depression or anger and you'll almost always find some frustrated desire or unmet need. Once you uncover the desire, you can deal with it. Face the desire, and you might see that it isn't all that important after all; then you can let it go. On the other hand, you might see that the desire is legitimate, something worth striving for. But if you don't even know what it is you really want, you'll continue to feel empty inside, devoid of fulfillment, and since you haven't a clue what the problem is and therefore don't know how to address it, you'll want to fill up the void with food.

My patient George stopped being angry and depressed the day he decided to go to law school. He no longer felt trapped being the accountant his father insisted he become.

Undoubtedly you've seen kids have a tantrum about not getting something that they wanted. Perhaps you thought, or even said to them, "Better start learning early that you're not always going to get what you want in life." Obviously, at this point in your life, it's no longer acceptable to throw yourself on the floor, scream, kick, and hold your breath when things don't work out according to your plan. You might *feel* like having a tantrum, especially when you try to fulfill infantile demands that are unrealistic, but it works much better to cultivate realistic, mature needs that you pursue appropriately, using realistic problem-solving techniques and making distinctions about how the world works. It is your responsibility to get your needs met appropriately within the context of your relationships, family, and work.

When you decide to fulfill a need, you have to balance your responsibilities, values, and loves, so any decision is by necessity a complex trade-off that only you can make. But when you engage in that complex trade-off you're operating in the real world of today, outside the domain of Harriet. That's your freedom space.

Linda decided to go back to school, though she also had a responsibility to be home for her kids by three o'clock. She knew that taking on the added pressure of getting her degree would make everything harder—managing the kids would be more difficult because of school, managing her schoolwork would be more difficult because of the kids, and overall she was afraid that managing her weight would once again fall to the bottom of her priority list. However, Linda was amazed at how creating a schedule and keeping to it made her more successful in all three of those areas.

How Harriet Keeps You from Fulfilling Your Needs

Sometimes your needs remain unfulfilled not because of outside circumstances, but because self-doubt makes you put on the brakes when it comes to trying to get your needs met. Because of Harriet, you feel that you don't have the capacity to get what you want, or that you don't deserve it, so you only make halfhearted or intermittent efforts to get it. Being blocked can make you resort to magical thinking, hoping that others will give you what you want or need without you having to ask for it. Perhaps you feel that it's too much of an imposition to ask for things—even things that you would be happy to give to others—as if you deserve less than others do. But waiting too long to be nurtured or respected or acknowledged or loved will make you hungry, both physically and emotionally. It will make you resentful, less likeable, moody, and fragile. And that will reinforce all your self-doubts.

The fact of the matter is that the people in your life rarely will satisfy your needs the way you hope they will, and too much hoping and wishing can leave you overly sensitive to disappointments. At the heart of your emotional hunger is a sense of hopelessness and a whole list of unfulfilled needs that you just can't seem to get met. This makes you eat more, in part because it makes you feel powerful and even hopeful, temporarily, to address a need you can fulfill—the need for delicious food.

Here's the conundrum. When you don't tell people what you want, you don't have a chance of getting it. And so you set up the people in your life to fail. They don't know what you want, and so they can't give it to you. And since you don't get what you want, you feel worthless and unloved; your host of unmet needs festers or grows; and you eat to comfort yourself, feel awful about pigging out, and then feel too unworthy to ask for what you need. So the cycle perpetuates and leaves you feeling like a loser.

Lilly is the mother at school who never says no. Lilly is a patient of mine who has been trying to lose thirty pounds for the last two years. Her four children go to a prominent Beverly Hills school and the teachers, the other mothers, and even the principal all know that Lilly will say yes to any committee, any play date, and almost every volunteer opportunity. At home, it's not much different. Her husband expects her to negotiate their social calendar and manage everything with regard to the children. Lilly says she's so busy she doesn't have time to think about what she needs, let alone eat properly or exercise. Getting your needs met takes real work. You may need to assert yourself, negotiate, make trade-offs, clarify communications, and maintain boundaries. You have to be willing to take a risk and put yourself on the line. If you experience sharp warnings from Harriet, doing this work might feel too anxiety-provoking: it might seem easier to simply ignore your needs—to repress them completely, or tell yourself you'll deal with them later. Again, the conundrum becomes that other people perceive you as someone who doesn't assert herself or himself and they run all over you, and you feel even more undeserving. But if you can believe that you'll survive even if your needs don't get met after you express them, if you're willing to take a chance, you have at least some possibility of fulfillment, plus you gain the self-respect of knowing that you stood up for yourself.

Facing Your Unfulfilled Potential

Avoidance sabotages our ability to have meaningful and truly inti-mate relationships. It undermines our clarity and creativity. It robs us of our capacity to be fully present in the moment. We think we are tuning out to avoid pain, but in the end, avoidance delivers us into the very pain, confusion, and unhappiness from which we are fleeing.—*Barbara De Angelis*

Another reason we don't fulfill our needs is because we fear failure if we attempt anything new. But no baby walks perfectly the first time, just as adults don't master equivalent challenges right away. And yet, stumbling, looking stupid, and failing frighten most of us so much that stagnation might seem preferable by comparison, and so we make the unfortunate choice to lay low.

Once you start avoiding challenges and abandoning your dreams, the road to the fridge is short. When you avoid challenges, you eat to stuff down frustration that comes from sitting on your own power. You eat to assuage guilt and sadness that your life isn't as full as it could be. You eat to avoid facing nervousness that comes from wanting to stay under the radar while also wanting to rise above it. You eat because you're torn between the self that you've always been and the self that you have an inkling you could become if only you'd take a risk.

What's so awful about the possibility of failing that you fear it with your whole being? Why rot and stagnate rather than take up a risky challenge? In order to stop the hunger-producing frustration and low self-esteem that come from avoiding challenges, you need to understand precisely what it is that you fear and what price you pay because of that fear.

Think about any mistakes you've made or humiliations you've experienced. How did you feel when you failed or made a mistake in public? In private? Don't forget the small mistakes or embarrassments, such as asking a "stupid question," or coming in last in a race.

My patient Catherine illustrates the price we pay when we fear challenges. Catherine had wanted to be a singer since she was a child. She still has cassette recordings of herself singing Madonna's "Live to Tell." She always felt free when she was singing. She was often asked to sing solos in the shows in her high school, but one day the boy she had a crush on made fun of her singing. She felt so humiliated that she stopped singing, except in her car when she was sure no one was watching.

When I asked Catherine about how she wasn't living out her dreams, she realized that she had abandoned something that gave her deep joy. Her dream was to make a living from her singing. The thing she immediately did was to start singing in front of people again. Catherine offered to sing at a friend's wedding. Her friends were surprised because they didn't even know that that beautiful voice was hiding beneath all of her weight.

The six-month goal I set with her was to make a demo tape. Catherine did this and used it to get a job as the music teacher at her local preschool. She no longer hoped to be Madonna, but by the time a year had rolled around she was working in a job where she was paid to sing. The children at the school loved her, and she finally felt fulfilled. Now Catherine no longer sits on the couch eating cartons of ice cream while watching *American Idol*; she's too busy learning songs to sing for her classes.

Perhaps, like Catherine, you've also given up old dreams. What was the end result of your mistake or failure? For instance, if you once had a terrible singing performance, did you stop singing? Or did you take lessons and improve? What does the way you handled your failure tell you? Have you avoided putting yourself forward in order to avoid the possibility of looking stupid again in public? What's the worst that might happen if you did look stupid? What is it that you fear? What opportunities have you missed by holding yourself back? How do you feel immediately after holding yourself back? What are the long-term effects?

If you actually spend a few moments thinking about these questions and possibly writing down your thoughts, you'll discover a very bad cold feeling in the pit of your stomach. Note it well. It's not pleasant, but it is bearable. It's your shame/fear condensed into a small compact space somewhere inside what seems like your gut, where it's easily converted into phantom hunger.

Please understand that the absence of a guiding dream creates an empty place inside you hungering to be filled up. You think a dessert or a plate of ravioli can give you a few moments of bliss, but no treat can substitute for a lifelong dream. When the food is gone, no matter how full your belly is, you're still empty.

Reclaim Your Dreams

> Keep on going and chances are that you will stumble on something, perhaps when you least expect it. I never heard of anyone stumbling on something sitting down.—*Charles F. Kettering*

Maybe you've determined that your dreams aren't meant for this lifetime, or that you can't fulfill them right now. You can't become a prima ballerina if you're sixty-five years old and arthritic, you can't make Timothy marry you if he already has a wife whom he loves, you can't go back to school full-time if you have no extra money and a dependent child. Perhaps, however, you can start taking the tiniest steps toward getting what you want. If you can't be a dancer, you *can* take ballet lessons. Maybe you'll find that tap dancing works better for you given your physical limitations, so you adjust your needs to meet the reality of your life. If you stick with dancing, who knows? Eventually you might form a troupe for senior dancers.

On the other hand, maybe you need to recognize that it's time to drop that particular desire to dance, to accept the frustration of dropping the dream and realize that frustration is a natural part of life. You need to assess what makes more sense for you—taking tiny steps to approach your dream, even if fulfilling that dream is a huge stretch at this point, or moving on to a new dream. If you choose the latter course, whether by choice or because you have no choice, you'll want strategies to help you navigate the frustration that comes with not getting what you want.

Here's the pep talk part of this session: True, failing might make you look stupid. If you aren't an expert, if you make mistakes, if you find out that you just don't have the necessary capacity, people may snicker and gossip—but you won't die from that. On the other hand, if you don't engage yourself in a dynamic process of trying new things, of chasing the challenges in your life, your spirit will, in fact, die, and you'll eat like a voracious lion besides.

As you undoubtedly know, the people who succeed most in life are those who endure failure well. If Edison hadn't failed ten thousand times, he never would have invented the battery. In fact, Edison turned fear of failure on its head by insisting that the more failures he had, the more likely he would be to eventually succeed. Jack London received six hundred rejections before he sold his first story, Henry Ford went bankrupt five times before he met with success, and Julia Child tried to sell her first cookbook for eight years before she found a publisher. It's no secret that cultivating resilience in the face of failure is a prerequisite for success.

What does this mean for you? You might not want to become another Babe Ruth or Henry Ford, but in the context of your own life, you have ample opportunity in which to cultivate an attitude of courage. The small events of everyday life present ample opportunity for developing resilience, for taking chances, for testing yourself, and for allowing yourself to grow in spite of the risks.

If you don't open up your latent potentials because self-doubt makes you fear failure and disappointment, then deep inside you'll feel like a coward, while the latent talent keeps calling out to you. You'll know that you haven't fulfilled your destiny or responded to new stages in your life cycle, and this perpetuates your self-doubt.

You have to at least try to fulfill your potential as much as you can in order to stop feeding your self-doubts. You have to take up at least some of the challenges in front of you, even though you might not ever realize your full dream. Or you have to make a conscious decision not to pursue your dreams because of other compelling considerations. But left in the murky no-man's-land of the unconscious, your failure to take chances and go for your dream remains a festering source of self-doubt.

Remember: if you don't find things to be passionate about in life, that creative energy that dwells within you will be forced into unproductive things like eating, arguing with your spouse, watching television constantly, and so on. Your life actually depends on you finding things that make your heart sing. Everyone has lists of things that they once dreamed about, everything from being president of the United States to flying to the moon to being a rock star. Some of those dreams may no longer be realistic, but let's revisit those dreams for the sole purpose of using them to create new dreams.

In part two, we'll look at your dreams and determine which ones are realistic to pursue and create new dreams. The story below about my patient Jess should illustrate how not following your dreams and taking risks affects your weight.

Jess Miller sat at her desk, staring out the window at the street below, watching a yellow cab cut off a Lexus. The Lexus honked, then pulled in front of the cab. "Great show," Jess said aloud.

In front of her, the annual report lay in a pile, waiting for her review, but she intended to put off reading it as long as possible. Everything about her job bored her lately.

"I need a new challenge," she muttered. Just as she reached for a cookie, her e-mail in box beeped. She had planned to ignore it, but then she saw that the message came from Dexter Norman, the CEO.

The message turned out to be a memo announcing that Jess's boss, Tom Winer, had resigned from his position as chief operating officer. Jess reread the memo three times. She wondered if Tom actually had been fired. Jess had liked her boss, but she knew Tom was incompetent. She also knew that she was next in line for the job.

The open position announcement came the next day. Jess got so nervous reading it that she made a trip to the kitchen for donuts and coffee before printing it out. She should apply, she knew, but she didn't have the MBA that the announcement called for, and so she wasn't qualified 100 percent. Plus, taking that job would put her in the firing line. She wasn't sure she was up to taking the heat. Did she really want to work that hard? Would she be up to the challenge?

For ten days, Jess equivocated, her donut quotient rising to four a day by the end of the application period. She just couldn't seem to get her materials together.

Two weeks later, another announcement arrived: Dina Leverton would be the next chief operating officer. She had applied right under Jess's nose and had gotten the job. Dina! Dina, who also had no MBA, who hadn't gone to Princeton, as Jess had, who wasn't half as smart as she was! How could Dina get the job that she should have gotten?

Jess boycotted the staff meetings that Dina ran for the next month, taking herself out to Starbucks during meeting time. When she found out that Dina had enrolled in an online MBA program, using her educational benefits, she examined the benefits packet to see if it was legitimate for her to use company money for online training. She briefly considered enrolling in the same program, but figured she shouldn't bother now.

For the next month, Jess continued to eat donuts daily. She put on 13 pounds by February and alienated the entire management team with her bad attitude. She told herself she should quit before she got fired, but just couldn't muster the energy to start the process of looking for another job.

Envy: The Great Informer

Jealousy is all the fun you think they had.—Erica Jong

As Jess Miller's story illustrates, envy provides a special way to avoid facing challenges. You can use envy to trick yourself into ignoring opportunities. Jess put her energy into resenting Dina instead of exploring her own inability to move her career forward. She actually hid behind envy, using it as a smokescreen to obscure her own dysfunctional behavior, her lack of willingness to take chances. She felt jealous of Dina simply because she had what she wanted, what she feared going after—not because she begrudged her success.

We naturally try to stifle jealousy because we've been taught that it's shameful, bad, ugly. And yet envy can be a great aid in the self-discovery process. If you don't know what you want, if you can't figure out what challenges you've been avoiding, envy has a message for you. Envy lets you know what you really hunger for— and it isn't food. In fact, envy delivers a message that you need to listen to carefully: envy tells you what you want, in no uncertain terms.

If you envy someone living a life that you wish you had, you need to pay attention to the buried message. That type of envy is loaded with the information you need about your deepest desires and frustrated hopes, just as Jess Miller's envy contained a clue about what she truly wanted—a go-getter attitude, courage to put herself forward, a more stimulating job.

Envy sends you a signal from within telling you that you want something more in life than what you have. If you try to suppress this signal by eating, you don't address your deeper needs or give yourself an opportunity to find satisfaction. And if you act out against the person you feel jealous of, your relationship ends up in the toilet, so you suffer even more in the end. Better by far to welcome the messages that jealousy brings and do something about them, making the requisite adjustments in how you live.

If You Can't Manage Your Stress, You Can't Manage Your Weight

The cause of stress is reality.—Lily Tomlin

There are certain things that you need to do to manage your life as an adult. You need to pay your bills and do your taxes. You need to get the oil changed on your car. You need to renew your driver's license and passport. You need to keep toilet paper in the house and take out the trash. They require some skill, but, more than that, they require discipline. When these things are not attended to, chaos reigns and you *might* feel scattered and incompetent. You feel like a fraud and end up hoping that someone will rescue you.

If you can't manage your day-to-day life, it makes it a whole lot harder to entertain the idea of going after dreams and goals. We have already established that addressing your self-doubts, cultivating satisfying relationships, and pursuing your dreams are critical components to ending your dependence on food as a reward. So let's look at ways that you can manage your life better so that you can feel confident and start doing some of the things that you'd really like to be doing. See if you see yourself in the anecdote below:

You're late for your meditation class. In your hurry to get there on time, you forget your wallet. Five miles down the highway, you realize that you're driving without a license, so you flip a U-turn and speed home. The phone rings.

"Ms. Jones," the nasal voice at the other end says, "you have a doctor's appointment today at two o'clock." You can't believe that you scheduled a doctor's appointment for the same time as meditation! Late for both appointments now, you frantically rip through the house searching for the wallet, which you can't find because you haven't cleaned in three weeks and everything is in a jumble. On the way to the bedroom, you grab a few cookies and shove them in your mouth without thinking. By the time you find the wallet in the pocket of yesterday's jeans, you're too late for either appointment, so you console yourself with more cookies and a mug of hot cocoa.

Does this sound familiar to you? Does stress make you desperate for a food fix?

Although you've probably recognized the connection between stress and the five-cookie syndrome before now, you might not have thought about what role food plays specifically in diminishing your stress. For one thing, food distracts you from the source of your anxiety, at least for a moment or two. That makes you feel better right away, but whatever has been making you anxious remains intact as long as you eat to forget about it, only to arise again as soon as the cookie crumbles in your digestive tract. Also, if you eat enough food, you go sluggish and dull, which might take the edge off the uncomfortable physical symptoms that anxiety causes, but again, the cause of the anxiety is still there.

Few things excite automatic eating the way that stress does. One minute you experience stress, and the next minute you've got a fistful of chips headed toward your lips, without stopping to think in between. Having too much stress increases the odds that you'll eat unhealthy food. Under stress, you tend to opt for food that won't take any more of your already frayed resources to prepare. You don't have the time to think about calories or health or even, necessarily, to cook something. Instead, you go to some fast food place or to the vending machine, or grab fistfuls of junk food off of your shelves.

My patient Laura illustrates the way stress can drive overeating. Laura is the single mother of Zachary, a five-year-old boy. She always wanted to be a mother, but didn't realize it would be this hard. Her husband left when her son was two months old and she has been on her own since. It would be one thing if her son were compliant; maybe then she would feel as if she finally had an ally in the world, but her son fights her on everything. By the time she manages to get Zach bathed and into bed at night, there are still so many things that need to be done. There are piles of dishes in the sink. There are stacks of unpaid bills. There is trash and recycling that need to be taken out. There is laundry. There are the cupcakes she has to make for Zach's class the next day. That doesn't even include all the things that she's been wanting to do for herself, the unread bestseller on her night stand, the single parents' event at the church, the online degree she's been looking at. She bakes the cupcakes because she wouldn't want to disappoint the teacher, eats four of them, and then just sits on the couch staring at the ceiling. She can't imagine how to begin to tackle everything that needs to get done.

Most of us, like Laura, use stress-reduction strategies that just don't work. Or they work for diminishing one type of stress, but not others. For instance, if you're stressed because you aren't making enough money, going salsa dancing won't necessarily help. On the other hand, if your stress comes from feeling ugly, the dancing might be just the thing. The trick is to isolate your current greatest stressors and find techniques that help you to get a handle on those things. You can begin by assessing the current techniques you use for handling stress, to see how they work for you. We'll work on this in part two.

Food May Be Your Friend, but It Won't Clean Your Closets for You

Nothing is so fatiguing as the eternal hanging on of an uncompleted task.—*William James*

There are two main types of stress: the stress that comes from acts of God or from circumstances that you have no control over, and the stress that comes from your own disorganization or from your personality issues. First let's talk about the stress that you create.

Like Laura in the story above, you might get so anxious about certain messes in your life that you just don't want to deal with them, which means that they get even worse. Much of the stress that grinds you down on a daily basis probably originates in your desire to steer clear of these unpleasant things. For instance, you want to avoid cleaning your fridge because it's such a disgusting mess that it makes you anxious to face it. Instead of tackling the science projects festering on the shelves, you go out to Wendy's for a burger and fries. The next day when you go to the fridge, the mess seems worse than it did before, and so your stress level goes up because cleaning it seems even more daunting than it did yesterday. And so it goes, to the point where you're going out all the time and the science projects grow legs and start walking. In the act of trying to avoid a little stressor, you've created a big one.

Creating order in your disheveled areas may help you to avoid the stress that leads you to get overwhelmed and eat. This means getting the tasks of daily life taken care of: paying the bills, doing the laundry, getting everything in order for your child's school. You need to clean your desk, do the taxes, get your doctor's appointments taken care of, go to the dentist, make the difficult call to Aunt Sally.

The avoidance that causes stress comes from an unconscious desire to circumvent adult responsibilities. To diminish this type of stress, you need to complete the developmental steps that will position you to face adult hassles head-on, instead of continuing to duck them like a child. For instance, if you experience stress because you can't say no to anyone and so have an overloaded schedule full of obligations, you need to take the developmental step of learning to say no. If you're stressed because your house is a wreck and you can't find anything, you need to learn how to create order in your environment. If you have outstanding calls to make, bills to pay, or reports overdue, you need to learn to complete administrative tasks on time, no matter how much you hate doing this. Unless you develop the competencies needed to negotiate everyday life, your self-esteem will suffer, and by now you know what that means for your diet.

It's one thing to avoid cleaning the fridge because you don't want to touch the slimy tomato mold, but quite another when you simply have no time for taking care of basic chores. When you work seventy hours a week and have classes at night, when you have eleven kids who belong to teams and clubs and need constant chaperoning, you've got a problem. Is the pressure that comes from being overloaded in the acts of God category, or is it self-imposed? And what can you do about it?

It's no secret that we've become a society of stress junkies. Many of us make choices that contribute to our ridiculous schedules—opting for high-paying jobs that demand our life blood, acquiring so much stuff that we have to work nonstop to pay for it and to repair it when it breaks down, frenetically running from activity to activity, not wanting to miss anything. Stress has become more the norm than the exception, and so you might even think it's desirable to be so scheduled-out that you have no time to take care of mundane tasks. But as you've seen, stress leads to ugly consequences, and so it pays to examine the choices you've made to see where you might create some space in your life.

Of course, you might have special sources of pressure that you can't control. Students in law school have to study around the clock, accountants during tax season have little time to breathe, unexpected financial crises might drive you to take a night job. But it's just as likely that you can free up enough time to get the laundry done, if you're willing to make some changes in your life. The bottom line is that if you say yes to making time for life maintenance, you need to say no to something else, and you have to be willing to do that.

Dara is a thirty-year-old online member who weighs 238 pounds. She never takes time to balance her checkbook, is always getting overdrawn, and infuriated her husband because as a result they now have a poor credit rating. She would rather ignore the checkbook than realize how little is there and get disappointed. She creates a lot of unnecessary stress for herself by not managing her time, and then when she's under stress, she always ends up bingeing.

Unexpected Sources of Stress

> Stress is not what happens to us. It's our response TO what happens. And RESPONSE is something we can choose.
> —*Maureen Killoran*

Some stress you just can't do anything about: things break, unexpected visitors appear, layoffs occur, illnesses arise, traffic happens. Maybe you have to work longer, harder, and with more interruptions than ever before—most of us do. Unless you've reached enlightenment or have supernatural powers, there's not much you can do to stop the assault of certain stressful events and circumstances.

So first you try to eliminate the stressor, if that's possible. If not, you try to handle stress in productive ways rather than trying to munch it down with fattening food. Instead of feeling victimized by your stress, recognize stress as an inevitable by-product of life on this planet, and understand that you have special equipment built into you for handling stress.

Some stress-busting techniques you probably know—taking yoga, going out for a run, practicing deep breathing, getting a massage. Other responses to stress might take a bit more creativity on your part. For instance, if you have excessive pressure at work, you might try taking a five-minute breathing break every hour. If you have an ill relative living with you, you might look into forming a support group. If you must drive in horrific traffic, bring books on tape with you.

To handle the stress in your life, it will help to analyze closely just what stressors impinge on you now, and brainstorm coping techniques before you find that food is your only answer.

Stress

When patients come into my office and their lives are clearly in chaos—they can't find their keys, they forget their checkbook, their check bounces not because they don't have enough money but because they forgot to deposit their paycheck—we look closely at ways for them to get organized. It is essential because until that happens, we cannot look at the deeper issues. If you live in chaos, Harriet is always there telling you, "Forget about solving your deeper issues; you can't even remember to bring the library books back on time."

If you feel victimized by the pressures on you, you'll probably fall into wild disorder. You remain stuck when you say things to yourself such as, "This pressure isn't fair, it shouldn't have to be this way, it's too much for me to handle." That's a way of you saying that you don't like reality and that you don't want to deal with it. And if you don't deal with it, you can't improve it.

SHRINK YOURSELF SESSION NOTES

You're the One Who's in Charge of Your Life

- You've learned that frustration with your life leads you to food as a reward.

- You've also learned that your frustration is based on a false sense of powerlessness, and that you have to recover your agency over your own life to master food.

- You'll have to make whatever changes are necessary to improve your relationships.

- You'll have to be the one who makes sure your legitimate needs get met, and your immature needs are given up.

- You'll have to take responsibility for your unfulfilled potential.

- You'll have to take charge of your stress, and improve the skills that make that possible.

- You must remember that you have two methods to recover your power over your own life:

  1. You can proactively deal with your life challenges and make your life work in the areas we've covered.

  2. You can avoid defeatism, adding to your false powerlessness, by not using obstacles and difficulties as justification to become a victim of your life, rather than the one in charge.

6

Your Safety Layer

I'm guessing that food still feels enticing, in spite of all the knowledge about shrinking yourself that you have so far—you just can't help yourself. Why? Because you're human—a complicated entity, full of contradictions. You say you want to lose weight and you have all the evidence to prove it—the diet books, the exercise videos, the low-fat foods in the fridge. *Unfortunately, you also have a part of yourself that wants to stay overweight.* This is different from what we've been discussing so far. Up until now we've been approaching this problem from the part of you that wants to lose weight but is having a hard time giving up the advantages of food as an over-the-counter tranquilizer. Now we want to look at a deeper layer, the part of you that *actually wants to be fat.* It's the part that is responsible for your regaining the weight after you've lost it, or the part of you that just digs in your heels and says, I just want to eat as much as I want, the hell with this diet stuff. We're introducing you to your rebellious self.

It speaks to the side of yourself that sabotages your efforts to diet, the part of you that wants you to stay fat—that actually uses your weight to prevent you from having the life you want. Most of this book has been dedicated to the rational side of yourself (the sensible self)—the you that's fully committed to losing weight, that wants to have a healthy and attractive body, better relationships, and life fulfillment. But this other part of you, which I call the rebellious self, not only resists your efforts to diet: it's terrified of losing weight. It's almost as if you have two beings inside at odds with each other. There is the part of you that desperately wants to lose the weight, and there is a part of you that sabotages all of your efforts.

Your rebellious self has two main modes of operation: either it cowers in the corner like a frightened toddler, sucking ice cream in spite of knowing better, or it acts out like a bratty kid demanding ice cream. In the first case it wants you to stay overweight in order to provide you a place to hide (under your fat), using weight as an excuse for not growing up or for avoiding romance and adult responsibility. In the second instance it wants you to stay overweight to assert independence from expectations or to get back at controlling people.

Everything you've learned in previous chapters has prepared you for doing this deeper exploration into the rebellious self. Now that you've learned that there are many adult alternatives for dealing with your moods and legitimate desires, you have everything you need to live better without using food as a short circuit or tranquilizer. Unfortunately, you also have the rebellious self to contend with. By bringing the reasons you honor the rebellious self into your full consciousness, you can think through whether or not you want to continue hiding behind your weight. Somewhere along the line you made a *decision* to use fat to avoid dealing with psychological and developmental issues. It might have happened when you were ten, or fifteen, or twenty, or even decades later. Now you have to make a new decision: do you still want to keep this protective layer of insulation, in spite of the cost to your health and happiness? Is it worth it?

What Does Fat Protect You From?

I feel about airplanes the way I feel about diets. It seems to me that they are wonderful things for other people to go on.—*Jean Kerr*

When my patient Joanne told me that being fat keeps men away, all of whom seem dangerous to her because of her background, I said to her, simply, "Aren't there better ways?"

Somewhere in the inner recesses of your psyche, you believe that you cannot provide safety for yourself out there in the big open world of your adult life, so you must find a place to hide, and you've discovered that being fat is a good place to hide.

Do you remember getting scared in childhood and hiding behind your parents? Or have you seen your own kids, or even your dogs, hide behind you when frightened? It's a natural human (and perhaps canine) impulse to seek shelter when threatened. For kids and dogs, the problem has an easy solution: cling to Mom's skirt or disappear behind Dad without disgrace. Once you grow up, though, the options narrow.

You might still feel the impulse to cling to someone when you feel threatened or uncomfortable, just like you did in childhood, but running behind Mom or Dad for protection at this point in your life just won't work. What options do you have? Either you need to face scary situations and people head-on, or you can develop a co-dependent relationship to disappear into, or you can hide inside yourself—literally.

Obviously, facing frightening things would be the healthier choice, but it's not necessarily the easiest choice. It might, in fact, be impossible if you are "sure" you are powerless to protect yourself when things get rough. We humans tend to opt for the path of least resistance. And so, in searching for the easy way, you might have discovered somewhere along the line that you could use your own fat as a metaphoric place to hide out—a kind of substitute for Mom's skirt.

Using food to keep you safe can start innocently as a delaying tactic: "I'll do it [look for a new job, pursue a relationship, go to the gym] when I lose ten pounds," and then you delay losing the ten pounds. You might have gone on to make your weight a way of retreating into your fat persona when danger threatened, using weight as an excuse for avoiding a host of challenges. And if excess weight has become your protective blanket, then getting thin means losing your security. If you're sure you're "powerless" to protect yourself, then it makes sense that you'd have a considerable investment in keeping the weight on.

You might be offended by the suggestion that you actually harbor the desire to be fat, especially given your ardent weight-loss efforts over the years. It may strike you as absurd to consider the possibility that there's a force inside yourself opposing the very rational goal of weight control that you've endorsed with your actions, your sweat, and your pocketbook. And naturally, your conscious mind would never drive you to choose fat over personal satisfaction. But how else do you explain your weight-control failures? The rebellious self operates deep inside the caverns of your mind. It might have germinated in childhood and taken root so quietly that you don't have any memory of actually deciding that being fat had its advantages. And you probably didn't actually make a conscious decision, although a few of my patients who were abused in childhood do remember exactly when they did make a deliberate decision to be fat in order to be unattractive.

I'm not making this up. I've seen repeatedly with thousands of patients and online clients how the rebellious self lures dieters back to fat over and over again with intimations of safety and rest. These patients all had a full commitment to weight loss—at least as far as they knew. But in the work of therapy, it became increasingly apparent to them, and to me, that something worked against that commitment—a force inside the psyche. And that force, it turned out, was a mistaken idea that being fat would somehow insulate the person from danger, hurt, and despair.

June, at twenty-three, couldn't stand her sister's envy any longer, so she hid in fat, ending the envy, but instead she was drowning in her own resentment about the sacrifice she had to make. Peter hid for the opposite reason. He was so successful at work that the pressure to be even better got to him. It was then that he discovered that when you are fat people no longer expect that much from you.

As long as some part of you still believes that being fat will make you be safe, you will always return to fat. It's human nature to return to safety whenever possible.

Your Logical Mind Knows Better

Your conscious, rational mind probably finds the idea of using food for protection an absurd notion. Most likely you consider fat a curse—not a warm, fuzzy blanket to snuggle inside, and so if you do, in fact, hide behind fat in order to protect yourself, chances are good that you haven't been aware of it. Chances are good that you feel uncomfortable with this material. But please don't take offense. Read on, and at least consider the possibility that you're a bit more attached to your fat than you care to admit.

Why might that unconscious of yours assume that being fat could make you safe? What shelter could extra weight possibly afford? As mentioned at the start of this chapter, being fat gives you an excuse to avoid uncomfortable sexual situations and sex in general. Also, you can use your weight to lower expectations, so that nobody expects too much from you. Fat gives you a reason not to go out, not to succeed, to have no love life—it provides a built-in excuse for virtually all endeavors. Plus, being fat keeps unwanted attention away. It prevents you from being in the same game as everyone else. It gives you a ready reason for not even trying in life. And if you don't even try, you're spared the pain of shattered dreams.

Let's explore more fully some of the ways that fat protects you.

Back in middle school, Lydia hated gym. She distinctly remembers one class during which she got selected to play on Alice Toma's softball team. Alice was the class jock, the girl everyone looked up to. Everyone wanted to be on Alice's team.

Up at bat, Lydia struck out. Then, in the field, she missed a fly ball.

"Idiot," one of her teammates yelled. "What a reject!" another chimed in. After school, two girls jumped her and hit her until she cried.

Gym became less of a problem after Lydia got fat. She never made it up to bat. Instead, she waited games out on the bench—the alternate who never got to play.

Like Lydia, you've probably had experiences when all eyes were on you and you blew it big-time. Remember the humiliation you felt? What could be worse? Few things cause excruciating psychic pain the way that humiliation and shame do. Even neglect doesn't hurt as much, at least not at the moment of occurrence. If in your past you suffered through a series of humiliations after putting yourself forward, you might have made an unconscious decision that you'd be better off laying low. So many of my patients and online members have told me how shy they were as children that I have come to believe that when the fat hiding place starts in childhood, it almost always gets triggered by shyness and shame.

As you know, in our culture, fat people get sidelined from the fast track. A recent National Association to Advance Fat Acceptance study found that overweight men pay a salary penalty of $1,000 per year per pound they're overweight, while 16 percent of employers admitted they wouldn't hire obese women under any conditions; an additional 44 percent would hire them only under certain circumstances. If prime-time television reflects popular sentiment, it's no surprise that a study at Michigan State University found that heavy TV characters are less likely to date, unlikely to have sex, and very likely to be the butt of bad jokes. Plus, they are rarely portrayed in leadership roles and often appear to have no friends of either sex.

We don't expect to see obese characters in the boardroom, the bedroom, or up on the big screen. And so when we meet someone significantly overweight, right away our expectations go down. We're less likely to expect heavy people to pull their weight, and we certainly don't expect them to excel. And so you can use fat in order to exempt yourself from career pressures, from relationship pressures, from the adult challenges of daily life. If you don't want to enter the fray, if you don't want to risk trying and failing, if you don't want to process the changes foisted upon you, you can circumvent these issues by keeping yourself fat.

The usefulness of fat as an avoidance mechanism covers a lot of territory. For instance, Fred, an online member, uses his weight to avoid facing the challenges of getting older. Fred says, "Being overweight gives me an excuse for looking flabby and sloppy. I need to face the fact that I'm aging, like it or not. I'm changing." Fred realizes that fat can't stop the aging process, although it can distract his attention away from it. Likewise, fat can't really save you from dealing with life, although it can give you a place to hide out while life gets even more complicated because of your negligence.

My patient Mary said, "I was a size 8 when I found out my husband was cheating on me. As many do, I blamed myself. I started eating to ease the pain, but also if I was fat that would be the reason he wanted someone else, not because I wasn't a good person. I ended up pregnant and we stayed together, but the damage was done. He had several other affairs and I continued eating after my daughter was born. I just gave up."

For Mary, eating was not just medication for her betrayal pain. She ate to be fat because fat protected her, just like a blanket of insulation, from the greater pain of thinking there was something wrong with her.

We've discussed the fact that others don't demand as much of you when you're fat, but there's also the reality that you might not demand as much of yourself—and that's the most pernicious effect of the rebellious self. When you're overweight, you can convince yourself that it's not worth trying to succeed because your fat condition won't allow you to compete. If challenges arise, you can excuse yourself completely or tell yourself, "I'll get to it when I'm thinner," or "First I have to lose some weight." That's a surefire way to stay fat. When you announce you're going to face a challenge you're afraid to tackle only if you lose weight, you're highly motivated not to lose the weight.

Again, it makes no logical sense to allow your weight to make you suffer just so that you can avoid the suffering that you might experience if you were to tackle life's challenges. And yet, somewhere in the hidden caverns of your consciousness, you've convinced yourself that the pain of being fat pales next to the pain of discovering your limitations. Plus, there's another fear that might drive you to the illogical decision to stay fat: not the fear of your own limitations, but the fear of life's limitations. It's one thing to fear that you'll let yourself down even if you do your best, and quite another to fear that life just can't give you what you want, that anything you achieve will ultimately bore and dissatisfy you. If you have a basic mistrust of life, staying fat affords you a way to keep from experiencing life's pleasures.

If you're staying fat so you won't be disappointed by your wishes and hopes not coming true, or at the prospect of not having the life you want, or because of the meaninglessness of existence, then you're depressed, and you're staying fat because of your depression. Depression saps all your energy, makes you tired, and makes dealing with the real world too much trouble, and not worth the effort. You're not just hiding, you're out of the game, you're in full retreat. By reading this, you might realize that perhaps you're not simply frustrated or disappointed, but you may actually be clinically depressed. If this is the case, you should seek professional help. In any case, though, the cure for depression involves taking charge of your life.

Sex and Fat

Perhaps you've had the experience of being pursued by someone whose advances you dreaded. Remember enduring that skin-crawly feeling of having someone breathing too close to you, crowding you, making you want to squirm away? Whether you were touched inappropriately as a child and developed an aversion to physical intimacy that still endures or had unpleasant encounters of the sexual type later on, including in the bedroom with your own spouse, you now find yourself in a quandary. On the one hand, you know that a primary marker of adulthood is engagement in sexual activity, and it isn't acceptable to tell your suitors or spouse that you're not in the mood for years on end. On the other hand, you find that you just can't stomach the intimacy. What options do you have other than working through the aversion and dealing with the consequences? You can opt for the priesthood or nunnery, or come up with a headache, or become so fat that you need no excuse because nobody wants to get close to you anymore.

In my practice, I see many people who hide behind their weight in order to avoid sex. My online client Lexy, for example, uses food to protect herself from early memories of trauma. "When Rex abused me," she writes, "I wasn't old enough to stop it or process the feelings, or figure anything out. I let the choice of becoming overweight happen. Because he was fat and ugly and I didn't want to touch him or be touched intimately by him, I think my ten-year-old mind assumed that if I became fat and ugly, he wouldn't want to touch me, either. It didn't work that way; it only generated painful contempt from others, but I didn't know how to find a different choice . . . I need to learn to be comfortable with the woman I am, graciously accept compliments and male appreciation, and know that as an adult, I'm capable of setting boundaries with others about how they may treat me, and enforce those boundaries. This would give me so much freedom from fear! Staying overweight allows me to continue hiding behind that ten-year-old's choice."

Lexy has a head start in resolving her problem because she recognizes where it comes from. She knows why she stays fat, at least in part, and so she can begin to dismantle the myth that fat will protect her. In her case, though, her difficulty originates from early, profound trauma, and so it will take some intense work to resolve.

More frequently, I see patients who use weight to protect themselves from issues popping up in their current relationships. My client Andrea, for instance, says her weight protects her from dealing with fear in her marriage and from acting on impulses that make her want to have an affair. She writes: "I have been using my weight primarily in my relationship with my husband. Continuing to overeat instead of taking action or risking rejection protects me. I thought that Ben was rejecting me for my weight, so staying that way gave me the illusion that [weight] was the only problem and that I wasn't the problem. I realize now that . . . if I want to stay in my relationship, I will have to change. I have to take charge of getting my needs met and not depending on him or blaming his rejection on my weight. [Plus] I have been afraid of being in an affair . . . because of Ben's lack of attention . . . so I have stayed fat to avoid this temptation. I'm rebellious against Ben, who blames his lack of attention to me on my weight. He's very materialistic, meaning how I look is an issue with him."

One of my patients was spied on by a sexual predator. She said, "I remember the day a stranger said something to me about my outfit. I started to eat to get fat, so no one would look at me like that again." To people like this patient, Lexy, and Andrea, extra layers of fat feel like protection from an unsafe environment or world.

Not every person who uses fat to avoid being looked at or approached by sexually aggressive people has had a real event to hang their discomfort on, but that doesn't make any difference. The discomfort can come from within and be just as strong, and often hardly conscious.

How Fat Becomes a Hiding Place

My weight is, I believe, one of the primary spiritual issues in my life . . . It is why I run from opportunities to lead and make excuses about my performance. . . . It's why I dread dressing up in a suit and being the adult I should be at my age and station. It's why I shy away from friendships, and project rejection on others. It's why I am painfully selfish. It's why I'm often grouchy, mean and overly sensitive for no reason. It's why I'm jealous of others. It's a source of resentment at God.—*Michael Spencer,* The Internet Monk

You could interpret Mr. Spencer's quotation above in two ways. First, you can think he is saying, "Because I am fat, I hide." On the other hand, he might be saying, "I stay fat or become fat in order to hide." The question is, which strategy resembles your own behavior?

You may be part of the first group. You became heavy for all the emotional eating reasons we have pursued in the preceding two sessions of *Shrink Yourself,* and because you're heavy, and embarrassed about it, you're hiding from the world until you lose the weight. But even if this is how it happened to you, once fat has become useful as a way of avoiding and hiding, the "I will do it after I lose weight" becomes a hiding place, just an excuse.

In essence, using fat to keep you feeling safe is learned and can be unlearned. You learned to use food to smother your self-doubts, to reward yourself when you felt defeated, and you also learned how to use food to keep you feeling safe. There's no gene that determines that.

You may have learned that being fat makes you feel safe when your father and mother divorced when you were eight, or when you were afraid of sex when you were fifteen, or when you went away to college and would rather order in pizza than face the cafeteria, or six months after you got married and things weren't going as well as you would've liked, or after your first baby was born and you felt isolated and overwhelmed, or after your children left the house, or during a separation from your spouse, or when menopause made you feel old, or when your parents died.

Once we stumble on the fat-as-protection solution, we find that it serves many purposes. One of the ways that many people use fat as a source of protection is to deal with their family dynamics. Probably the best way to explain this is to remind you of the importance of roles in families. Think back on your own extended family. One sister or brother was the athlete; another the brain; the third the dramatic one. Then there was the one destined for success; the beauty; the hunk; the black sheep; the angry one; the rejected and unloved one; the favored; the alcoholic; the bad-tempered one; the oversexed one; the bad student; the shy one; the stubborn one; the ugly one; the caretaker. You and everyone you know fit some role stereotype like these while growing up. These assigned roles are our family legacy and control much of what we do and how we think about ourselves until the time we emerge from them. Most of us do emerge completely over time, but some don't. When fat is used as a hiding place, the emergence can't occur.

Family-assigned roles distort who you are and limit who you're capable of being. And they are all accidents of life, the consequence of converging forces beyond the control of anybody. If you had been born the oldest instead of the youngest, you might have been the black sheep instead of the favorite. If your mother liked herself better, or married differently, or later, or to a different husband, you might not be as angry as you are or as much of a people-pleaser as you had to be.

If you were a seriously overweight girl, it might have gone something like this: when in the grips of any of these roles, you might have discovered fat as a way of coping. You couldn't compete with the beautiful sister, so you had to be the rejected one. Being fat gave that role the support it needed, justified the envy you already felt toward your sister, and at the same time paid back your parents for their unfair treatment and misunderstanding of you by forcing them to agonize with you about your unpopularity at school. Once this dynamic was established it fed on itself, and your psychological conflicts at home became embedded and enshrined in your fat identity.

Real versus Imagined Safety

The real danger of stepping out of a family role and reclaiming yourself is the danger of being punished, ostracized, and envied by others. You fear being talked about, labeled, excommunicated from the clan. When you lose weight and become intent on remaking your life, you expose yourself to these ancient anxieties, and the rebellious self tells you that you can feel safe again only if you will get fat again.

You can see how the buffering that fat provides might hook you into staying overweight, although, of course, fat doesn't really protect you. You know it doesn't make logical sense to try to hide behind fat, given the fact that excess weight is seen as unattractive, and that it's harmful to your health. At one time in history, being fat meant you were prosperous, and even as late as the turn of the last century there were clubs designed to fatten up young ladies so they would appeal to prosperous mates. But that story has changed, and you know it has. Your logical mind knows it makes no sense to stay fat, and knows the cost you pay for staying fat.

And so on the one hand you have the illusion that fat will keep you safe, and on the other, the reality that fat actually makes you very unsafe, physically, economically, socially, and emotionally. It's time to recognize that fat only makes you feel safe but doesn't bring you real safety, so you can decide that you are paying too high a price for an illusion. The first step is to make the distinction between real safety and the illusion of safety.

The main distinction to keep in mind is that the illusion of safety is really the illusion of absolute safety. That is, while in the grips of the illusion of safety, you think nothing can go wrong. It's a very seductive idea. It's the deepest wish of an anxious child or adult. The idea of absolute safety represents the opposite of all of our fears about what might happen to us, physically and emotionally. The illusion of absolute safety is what makes the food trance so comforting when we go into the escape bubble. Perfect safety is the goal of the heroin addict as well as the alcoholic who drinks him- or herself into a stupor of oblivion. We will do anything for absolute safety—for the possibility of living a life where nothing or no one can harm us.

Real safety, on the other hand, is always relative safety, since in the real world there is no absolute safety. Tomorrow your routine bloodwork taken during your annual physical can be the beginning of a fight to survive. Your friend or relative may die of a heart attack. A good business can go sour. A secure job can be lost. Your child can have an accident. A great relationship can turn into a nightmare. You can increase your real safety in the world by facing reality, looking for real dangers, anticipating problems, and looking for solutions. You can keep your relationships strong, and invest yourself in good people who are trustworthy and decent and well put together. You can avoid impulsive big decisions like falling in love and marrying before you really know the real person, or marrying the wrong person to spite your parents. There are hundreds of things you can do and skills you can further develop to provide yourself with as much safety as possible in what is at times an unpredictable world. But to be your own adult provider of real safety, you have to face reality, whatever it is, and work with it. When you hide in fat to give yourself the illusion of safety by avoiding challenge, you are not facing up to reality, and are missing the opportunity to take charge of your own safety and make it as real as possible.

Fat doesn't bring you any real safety. In fact, it makes you less safe because you aren't creating your own real safety by dealing effectively with the challenges and opportunities of your life. If you apply only a half-mindful effort to your career or marriage because you want to avoid certain pieces of psychological work or difficult decisions, if you hide behind fat in these arenas in order to "duck out," your marriage and your work will be less likely to continue successfully in a way that's satisfying.

You believe that fat provides safety based on the illusion that you can buy time before you have to face the imaginary firing squad. Avoidance, fat, and the illusion of safety work together, reinforcing one another, and that is why fat is such a good hiding place.

Using fat this way is also a way of fooling yourself. You are not admitting to yourself that you have made certain decisions about the way you are now conducting your life. For instance, if you are using fat to avoid being sexually involved, then you have made a decision to not be sexually involved. Why not just accept that as fact, and either stick to your decision (it is your right and your body), or reevaluate your decision and work on your fears? Either decision would be more clearly adult, and would make you a more powerful person. But using fat to avoid sexuality makes the whole decision process muddy.

If you don't want sexual attention, just say no, or dress conservatively, or stay away from bars and discos, or send out signals to your boss that you're unavailable.

If you're shy, either work on it or accept it. Plenty of shy people do that without having to be heavy to call attention to themselves, which is the opposite of what most shy people consciously want.

If you don't want to have affairs or be promiscuous, either decide to remain monogamous and stick to your decision, or figure out why you're looking outside your relationship, or why it feels impossible to remain committed.

If it's intimacy, success, failure, or competition you fear, deal with it or live with it; there's no need to add fat to the equation. These are separate life course decisions that you have to make, or have already made, that end up getting more complicated when you add fat to the mix. They need to be separated out and dealt with for what they are, not covered over and buried by food and fat cells.

It's better to own up to the decision and not be fat. Then you have only that one problem to resolve. Fat doesn't protect. It only covers over a decision already made, and prevents an honest review of that decision. It keeps you stuck. And being stuck means you are at least temporarily powerless.

One of the online members of Shrink Yourself said, "Once I realized that I was in a thirty-eight-year marriage that was going nowhere and made the decision to leave, the fat just became a useless blanket I was hiding beneath." This almost-300-pound woman had used fat as a place to hide out from the fact that her marriage was a disaster since the first day, but she didn't want to admit it to herself. If she had not hidden that awareness under fat, she might have made a decision a lot earlier and started over with someone new when she was twenty-five and thin rather than facing the much tougher challenge of finding a mate at sixty-three, with a lot of loose skin to hide. The illusion of safety provided by fat cost her dearly because she forfeited the opportunity to provide herself real safety by making a better decision about staying married to a man with a severe and intractable alcohol problem.

Hiding behind fat is a real contradiction. People who are seriously overweight or morbidly obese hate the fact that they're discounted and misunderstood, or looked down on as weak-willed or lazy or gluttonous. They hate the fact that they're romantically "invisible" or thought of as "not in the game" or not considered to be potential leaders or desirable co-workers. But everything they hate about this stigma is what they're using as protection. They eat themselves into the stigma, then use the consequences of the stigma as their protective covering. They use the fact that they are not in the romantic game or expected to be too successful as an excuse to avoid those challenges.

And of course the stigma only adds to self-doubts both directly and indirectly. Directly, because no human can totally ignore or discount what others think of him or her. We are social animals who are programmed to attend to and care about what others think of us. Indirectly, being stigmatized puts us at war with, and alienates us from, those who misunderstand us. That means that we carry a load of chronic anger that feeds our doubts about our essential goodness.

So all of our logic and good sense tells us that fat doesn't make us safe in any real way and that all we get in return for the extra pounds that will shorten our lives is an illusion that lets us avoid continuing the essential work of human development. Not a very good bargain, if you ask me.

SHRINK YOURSELF SESSION NOTE
Create Your Own Sense of Safety

- You'll have to face your anxiety instead of eating to give yourself the illusion of being safe or independent.

- You'll have to do the grown-up work in the real world that could actually get you real safety and real independence.

- You'll have to stop reinforcing your self-doubts by avoiding something important, the grown-up work.

- You'll have to realize that your self-doubts make you more dependent, anxious, and sensitive to failing and embarrassment, and make you look for a hiding place.

- You'll have to see how you eat more to *feel* safe, but it doesn't *make* you safe, it just helps you avoid things and keeps you from recognizing the life decisions you've made that should be reviewed.

- You'll see that there are better ways to deal with the challenges you're hiding from other than using fat as a cover-up and excuse.

- You know that you have two methods to dismantle the false conclusion that you're incapable of providing your own safety in life:

  1. You can use these insights to stop hiding so you can discover for yourself that you're not powerless.

  2. You can stop misinterpreting the dangers in your daily life in order to stop reinforcing your conclusion about powerlessness.

7

Your Rebellion Layer

The man in one *New Yorker* cartoon says, "I became a vegetarian for health reasons, then for moral ones, now it's just to annoy people." If you've ever announced new dietary preferences to your family, you might have experienced something similar. Perhaps your so-called loved ones acted annoyed or even threatened when the subject of your new diet came up, as if by changing your diet, you were abandoning the family. One of our online members says, "Even when I tell my mom that I'm watching my weight, she still prepares all of my favorite fattening foods. It's almost like she doesn't want me to lose weight."

Kids discover early that if they don't eat according to parental guidelines, their parents become agitated. If you didn't eat your broccoli, Mom got anxious. If you ate too much broccoli, Mom worried. If you threw broccoli into the orange juice, Mom got furious. Your child mind observed all of this and recognized that Mom's moods altered depending on how you handled food. Translated, that meant that if you wanted to control Mom, you could alter what or how you ate. By overeating or by eating junk food, you could act out without throwing a temper tantrum, without posing a direct challenge, without putting yourself in the line of fire. Although you were controlled by your parents, you learned how to counterpunch, which at least gave you some feeling of powerfulness.

Kids naturally look for some avenue by which they can assert their power, because they have so few options. As a kid, you had no freedom, no real voice in what happened to you. Learning to say "no" in the terrible two's is a developmental milestone of individuality and autonomy. By playing with your food, by overeating, by gorging or sneaking sweets, and in some cases by not eating, you discovered that you could assert your autonomy in a semiacceptable way. Simply by eating, or by refusing to eat, or by constantly nagging for food, you could exasperate Mom and get her attention! Or you could trump her authority by sneaking food behind her back.

If you now have children of your own, you will be quite familiar with this pattern. You tell your children not to do something and you know they understand what you're saying, yet a second later they do the exact thing you just prohibited. "No more candy, Joey," you say. Joey waits until you turn your back and then grabs a fistful of Gummi Bears. You simply can't understand why he would want to get into trouble over and over again. Doesn't he know that he would have so much more fun if he just complied?

That part of you that wanted to spite *your* parents, that wanted to prove that you could do it your own way, hasn't gone away completely. Sure, you have to keep it in check to some degree or you wouldn't be able to maintain any relationships or hold down a job, but a part of you still wants to do it your way at all costs, because the pattern, once established, becomes entrenched. Though it might be relegated to your unconscious mind, it still plays the old tape, which goes something like this: "They can stop me from doing everything else, but I retain the power to eat as much as I want, and to eat what I want. I'll sneak or binge and purge or do anything necessary to keep this basic building block of autonomy."

So you still have this rebellious pattern, except the object of your rebellion has long since disappeared. Your parents no longer control what you wear, what you say, or what you eat. Now you're acting out against your own critical conscience, in other words, Harriet.

If you're still rebelling against your own conscience with food, it's a sure sign that in this sector of your mind, you haven't evolved past your primitive struggle against your parents' control. You're still stuck with this indirect and now ineffective and self-destructive way to assert yourself because you still believe that you're not allowed to express appropriate aggression or confrontation when it is called for in your adult life, and this is especially true if the one you need to confront is your parent or a spouse or a boss. You're still being held back by your primitive assessment that your anger is bad anger, and can't ever be a good and useful source of power. You still view yourself as a dangerous time bomb about to explode and injure, rather than a person coping with life. These assessments make you feel powerless, and hungry to act out your aggression in the only place you dare, onto yourself. One patient said, "I put food in my mouth to keep me from spitting out angry words."

You act out against yourself. You express your defiance by eating. No one is going to tell you what to do. Obviously, this approach to asserting yourself lacks logic. But it is a normal behavior and I see so many people do it. Instead of autonomy, you display self-destructive behavior. It may give you a false feeling of being in control to eat as you please, just as it gives toddlers a feeling of control when they throw food or refuse to eat broccoli or scream for candy. Defiant food control is the mechanism of choice for the terrible two's, but hardly a rational choice for adults.

Before we move on, scour your memory to see if you can recall any times in your childhood when you used food to assert your autonomy. Did you ever sneak food? Did you refuse to eat or refuse to stop eating? Did you know you were being disobedient in doing so? Try to recall the emotions you experienced. Was there any sense of doing what *you* wanted in spite of what "they" wanted?

Instead of using fat as an immature way to express hidden aggression, you must learn the skills of expressing appropriate and useful aggression as well as admitting when your anger is unjustified and needs to be curbed, or apologies need to be made.

Several of my patients have told me that they eat "at" people, meaning that when in a restaurant with friends who are watching how much they eat, they purposely eat much more than they want as a metaphoric way of saying what they don't want to say in words.

Six Ways You Use Food to Rebel

As you know, the angry rebellious self gets activated for a variety of reasons and acts that anger out through food and eating. Some people didn't get the independence or nurturance they needed early on, and now they assert their will, or test the love coming to them, by eating in opposition to the demands of others. Some people eat because they want attention they didn't get, and they know wanton eating can do the trick. In some cases, the defiant self just stonewalls the expectations and demands it finds offensive.

In almost all cases the aggression itself is masked and disguised. Here are some of the most common theme songs of the rebellious self:

1. Love me first, then I will lose weight.
2. They made me this way, so I can't change.
3. I'll get back at them.
4. I'm not this body.
5. Food is the only pleasurable thing I have, so I'm not giving it up.
6. If I can't be perfect, I'd rather be fat.

Let's look at each of these agendas in depth and see if any of them apply to you.

1. Love Me First, Then I Will Lose Weight

My patient Darlene grew up in a one-parent home. Her mother had to work two jobs to keep the family afloat, and Darlene often stayed with relatives. Her mom came home from work late, then cleaned the house, took care of the bills and the laundry, and tended to her own sick mother. Darlene felt abandoned and comforted herself with junk food. By age six, she had already started putting on weight.

Now she's twenty-four years old, and Darlene has a boyfriend who recently suggested to her that she lose weight so that they can be more active together. Darlene reacted by eating herself sick at the Marriott buffet the next morning. Darlene's rebellious self didn't want to be judged because of her weight. Instead, it demanded unconditional love no matter how she looked or what problems her weight caused—the sort of love she had missed as a child. The motto of her rebellious self was, "Love me first; then I will lose weight."

Darlene neither recognized her boyfriend's genuine concern for her, nor acknowledge the legitimacy of his desire to enjoy activities with her. She was so caught in the old tape loop of feeling neglected and unloved that she couldn't see the current reality. Her boyfriend became the spitting image of her critical conscience, which was the spitting image of her depriving mother. Her rebellious self still fumed that she didn't get the love and protection that she needed as a child, and that made it difficult for her to accept the love that came to her later in life.

Like Darlene, if you experienced early deprivation, you're probably wary of any love that comes your way. Even when Prince (or Princess) Charming shows up, instead of rejoicing, you spend your time worrying that he's actually a frog. Instead of accepting love and giving love back, you test and retest Prince Charming, perhaps by getting fat.

"If he really loves me, he'll see that under this fat I'm really a princess," says your rebellious self. "First he has to love me—he has to kiss me as the frog, and then I'll lose weight and show my true self."

The rebellious self holds that if Prince Charming—or the relevant friend or colleague—really loved you in the right way, they would accept you as you are. Then you would lose the weight. You've set up a test, an assessment of the other person's love for you. And in so doing, you try to convince yourself and everyone else that the way you look is fine and that they should accept you, flaws and all. It's a no-win game for you because if you lose weight for him and he enjoys your new body, then you think that he only really loves you when you are thin, so you punish him for admiring you by gaining the weight back.

Obviously, this way of thinking has little merit, because if you stay fat, Prince Charming might get exasperated and actually turn into a frog himself. He might get fat or just leave you because you look bad and you don't trust him. Meanwhile, you're killing yourself using your own body as a battleground for old hurts that don't apply in your current situation. Who gets hurt the most? Not the person who initially withheld love from you, and not the person trying to love you now (because he or she can go on to find other love). You get hurt because when you use your body in this way, the battle takes a toll on your health, your happiness, your chances for love and intimacy, your self-esteem, and your energy.

Think about this: if you expect your dear ones to love and accept you as you are, you must do the same for yourself. How do you feel when you look in a mirror? Do you believe your body is fine as it is? Are fat folds really beautiful? Isn't the natural shape more inherently attractive? You can't convince yourself to ignore the fat, so you spend your life energies trying to convince the people in your life that they should. It's a no-win, dead-end, wasteful game. Think about the logic.

The real you, the person who wants the love, lives inside the fat, underneath it. Isn't that the part of yourself that you want to share with those who love you?

Read this letter from an online member:

My question revolves around how to get over deep-seated feelings of being inferior physically. This started at around age 8. A few incidents of being teased at school have stuck with me. Kids would tease me by chanting, "Do Re Mi Fat So La Ti Do." I was passed over at parties when we played spin the bottle, and shopping in the chubby section took its toll. By the time I reached my teens, I was afraid to compete with other girls and I felt unattractive to boys.

This has continued all of my life. I married very young to

the first and only person I've ever had sexual experience with. Although his relationship with me has improved my self-esteem, I still see my own lack of self-esteem as the biggest weight issue. Can you provide any advice?

This member is sixty-two, still at that party where they're passing over her during spin the bottle. She doesn't see the man in front of her hoping the bottle lands on him. What she tells me in other parts of the program is that she has been punishing her husband with her fat for other things, using her body as a battleground in her current life, prolonging and reinforcing the childhood wounds. She doesn't let him look at her or touch her, even though he says he's attracted to her just the way she is. She's right that self-esteem is her biggest weight issue, but what she has to realize is not just that something happened in growing up to create her inferior feeling, but that she is perpetuating it unnecessarily, and that she can reverse it (not the memories) by finding a much better dialogue with her husband than through letting her fat talk, and stop looking at him as just like all the other boys from the past.

She needs to have a real love affair with herself rather than continue seeking the unconditional love that no one ever gets for very long. It's holding out for unconditional love that keeps the angry furnace burning bright, and that makes your anger dangerous.

2. They Made Me This Way, So I Can't Change

If you could kick the person in the pants responsible for most of your trouble, you wouldn't sit for a month.—*Anonymous*

So often I hear people say they were made fat by the way they were brought up. My client explains, "We were a family of four but my mother cooked for twenty. Spaghetti, ravioli, greasy garlic bread, the fattiest foods. I always had to finish everything on my plate and then there were seconds and thirds, and always desserts. No wonder I'm fat." Another tells me, "We're a fat family. What can I do? Everyone overeats in my house."

Those who don't blame childhood mealtime for their weight problems sometimes say they became fat because they received so much criticism of their appearance as children that they couldn't handle it. They got fat because they had to escape the constant surveillance of how they looked, or because they received so much criticism after putting on weight that they became paralyzed into inaction.

Of course, the meal habits of your family did affect your weight as you matured. If you grew up a fat kid, or if early on you learned poor dietary habits, it might be more difficult to lose weight as an adult. There may be much historical truth to support the claim that your early experience contributed to making you an overweight adult: it might even be the main factor. But as the saying goes, the past is dust. If you put all the blame on the people who raised you, you remain stuck in the past, as powerless as you were back then.

Perhaps you don't blame your family of origin, but you point to your current spouse or partner or roommates. Someone in your household cooks too much or brings junk food home, or tempts you to go out to eat too often, and you end up paying the price. Blaming your friends and loved ones now is just a variation on the "blame the family" game. Instead of placing blame, why not consider what role you play in making food choices at home?

In order to move forward, you have to shed the victim role, even if it fits you as comfortably as an old pair of sweatpants. Instead of wallowing in blame and regret, why not focus on what you have working for you now?

I had a patient who begged for piano lessons every day since she was three. Her parents told her that they wouldn't get her a piano because she would probably get bored and give it up. As an adult, she has spent a lot of time angry that she doesn't know how to play the piano. When she feels angry, she puts on piano concertos and eats chocolate. It's true that she may never be as good as if she had started lessons at three, but blaming her parents doesn't make her a piano player—it just keeps her angry.

Compare her story to that of Emmanuel, a young man from Ghana featured in the documentary *Emmanuel's Wish*. He was born with only one leg, into a poor family, in a country where disabled people like him were shunned. In fact, his father was so ashamed of his son that he deserted the family after Emmanuel's birth. Then his mother died when he was thirteen, and Emmanuel had to drop out of school to support his family by shining shoes for two dollars a day.

Instead of sinking into blame, despair, and anger, Emmanuel maintained a dream that he would ride a bicycle across his country to prove that disabled people could rise above their deformities to do amazing things. He managed to contact a funding agency in the United States, get a bike, complete his ride of six hundred miles using his one leg, and then worked to better conditions for all disabled people in his nation. At this point, Emmanuel has become a national hero, has met with the secretary-general of the United Nations, has won many athletic awards, and has helped thousands of people in his country move from begging to productive careers.

The not-so-hidden anger embedded in this type of rebellion goes something like this: "You did this to me. You should've been a better parent and anticipated how the way you treated me would affect me and my weight. If you had been this perfect protective parent I deserve, I wouldn't be this way. I'm not going to do all the work of fixing what you did to me by taking control of my weight and letting you get all the credit."

As Emmanuel's story shows, with attitude adjustment, success can bloom from the most unpromising background. If you know that you blame others for your weight problems, you might ask yourself if you're more committed to placing that blame or to having the life you want.

3. I'll Get Back at Them

> A man that studieth revenge keeps his own wounds green.
> —*Sir Francis Bacon*

Some people who didn't get the love they wanted during childhood are still having a temper tantrum about it well into adulthood. Their rebellious self feels satisfied with nothing short of revenge.

One of my clients, a thirty-nine-year-old woman named Nancy, recently told me, "I stay overweight as a way to let my mother know that she failed me when I was a child by not teaching me good eating habits and boosting my self-esteem. I ended up overweight just like she did. So, by being overweight, I guess [I'm] subconsciously shoving it in her face by not losing the weight. I'm proving to her that I'm fat and damaged and that she should have been there for me as I was growing up."

If Nancy's story resonates with you, you have seething anger at one of your parents. This parent became your enemy way back in the ancient history of your life. He or she was supposed to love and protect you, to encourage and understand you. Instead, something else happened, and you haven't forgotten it. You have a giant score to settle. Even if that parent now feels guilty and makes sincere attempts to apologize, your anger doesn't abate. Even if that parent has already died, the fury still festers inside you. You feel wronged, that you were damaged in some permanent way, and you're stuck with this need to get even.

My patient Diane lost her mother five years ago, but she still shakes with rage when she thinks about her. Diane made a decision years ago to spite her fastidious mother by gaining weight. She feels that her mother deprived her in every important way, preferring her sister, withholding affection, insisting on academic perfection, caring more about what the neighbors thought than about Diane's needs, striking Diane on occasion. Diane circumvented her mother's control by getting fat, and she remains fat in defiance.

It might be important for Diane to disavow her mother's treatment of her, but there's a big difference between standing against mistreatment and shutting the door to relationship if the other person can't act with civility, versus staying in a rage because of that mistreatment. Diane certainly can't hurt her dead mom by staying fat herself. The rage that she harbors keeps peace, success, and satisfaction always at bay for her.

Unlike Diane, not everyone who stays overweight to get revenge has issues with their family. Sometimes people want to get back at someone in their life now—a child, a rejecting lover, a spouse. I have a patient who wants her husband to stop smoking because she has asthma. He quits for a while and then starts again. Each time he takes up smoking, she puts on forty pounds to punish him. What message does this send to her husband about how much she *really* values her own health?

You'll never win the battle by using your body for revenge. You might not want to let the perpetrator get away with hurting you, but it doesn't help to hurt yourself. Better to stop perpetuating past pains that should be long over. Better also to communicate with anyone in your life now who angers you, so that you might actually transform the relationship and find satisfaction in it. Or if you discover that there's no hope of reconciliation, better to move on with your dignity, and body, intact.

Remember what you learned in World History class: revenge tends to be self-sustaining. Once a nation or a tribe establishes a grievance, they'll blindly fight for restitution generation after generation. Likewise, if you have grievances that started decades ago, you may still be fighting inwardly, holding onto horror stories that you've never revisited for accuracy or meaning, feeling yourself to be the victim of a huge injustice or hypocrisy, interpreting your own experience with the same mind-set you applied at age four. It's time to stop using your bulging belly as a billboard. Nobody is interested in the secrets you are trying to expose.

4. I'm Not This Body

> Survivors commonly speak of how they endured trauma by pretending that their mind and spirit had gone to a safer place, leaving the body behind to endure the abuse.—*Skittles Place*

When Sara was ten, her father asked to come in and watch her shower. Sara felt she was old enough to shower alone and the idea of it made her feel uncomfortable. Her father insisted and finally, feeling guilty, she gave in. As he stood there, she psychically left her body, splitting herself off from the person in the shower so that she didn't have to own the shame she experienced. Later, when her father developed the habit of kissing her good night on the lips in a lingering way, she perfected the art of taking flight. Her body remained in bed, but the rest of her went to a safe garden that she created in her imagination.

Likewise, Barbara's mother flew into rages during which she assaulted Barbara, hitting and kicking her. Her mother's dark moods came on without warning, and when they did, anything that Barbara said or did could result in a physical attack from Mom. Barbara, too, dissociated from her body during the attacks. *She can strike me on the outside, but not on the inside,* Barbara told herself. Meanwhile, she left her body behind to fend for itself.

The habit of dissociating from the body became so entrenched for these two women that they barely noticed when they gained weight. They didn't "live" inside their bodies enough to care. Sara hasn't returned to her body fully since that day in the shower, and now she's 80 pounds overweight. Barbara weighs 45 pounds more than she should.

Like Sara, many children had devastating attacks on their body through harsh punishment or sexual predators. To escape the pain, the shame, and even the confusing feelings of arousal, they dissociated just as Sara and Barbara did. This type of dissociation really happens. If you've suffered abuse, perhaps it's happened to you. Ask yourself if you fully live inside your skin. Do you often have feelings of floating, of being "spacy?" Does your body feel like a foreign entity sometimes, separate from the real you? Do you ignore your body's signals and needs? If so, you also have learned to dissociate.

Continuing to pretend you have no body or no responsibility for your body is an illusion that keeps you from being a unified being, a person capable of finally keeping yourself safe from harm. You can pretend you have no body to yourself, but your mind and body know differently. Everything that happens in your body is known by your mind. It's not another person who binges at 2:00 A.M. You may need to get some special help in overcoming trauma in order to merge back into your physical being. Getting that help from a trained mental health professional who specializes in trauma can help you to overcome depression, apathy, and a host of other seemingly unrelated issues.

5. Food Is the Only Pleasurable Thing I Have, So I'm Not Giving It Up

While you might think the declaration that food offers your only comfort smacks of pathetic, pitiable sadness, it actually broadcasts defiance. You tell the world that you can't find any other option, that you don't enjoy the gifts others offer, that life stinks, and so you'll take care of your own needs, no thanks to anyone else. In other words, the position reeks of anger, of an exaggerated snit. It's just another example of rationalizing the decision to eat in order to rebel.

It's just not true that you have no choices and no life to live and no real path to legitimate pleasure in life. Your life is full of possibility. It is not so difficult, no matter what you are facing, to honestly believe that you have more reasons for living than the promise of one more full stomach.

6. If I Can't Be Perfect, I'd Rather Be Fat

This agenda suggests that the only position worth having in life is being the winner. And if you can't be the winner, then why bother playing the game? It is a childlike way of thinking. It renders any small improvements in your weight, your shape, your mobility, and your breathing unimportant.

Two Mistakes That Keep You Rebelling

Mistake # 1. Rebellion Is Not the Same as Independence

> Better a hundred enemies outside the car than one inside.
> —*Arabian proverb*

By now, perhaps you've begun to see how the rebellious self drives you to use food as a substitute for autonomy. With luck, you also can see how irrational it is to use food in this way. Your twelve-donut-a-day habit will never lead you to the one person who will love you the way you wanted to be loved when you were seven, because now you're twenty or thirty or fifty—and fat. It won't punish the people who hurt you in your past and it won't make you free from them, either—you're already free and independent and grown up. You no longer need to eat recklessly to prove to anyone that they can't control you. They can't!

When you put that food into your mouth, you probably don't think, *Ha ha, Mom. I'll do it MY way. I'll eat what I want . . . so there!* No. You just see the food and it smells great and you want it. But under the surface of your consciousness, the rebellious mechanism plays out, driving you to eat foolishly in spite of your higher reason, in spite of your health, in spite of your diet. You eat how you want, and nobody can stop you.

The first mistake you make that keeps the rebellious self in place is confusing this feeling of defiance and rebellion with true independence and autonomy. I think you have seen that difference illustrated quite well here, but it'll be up to you to keep that distinction in mind, and be sure to label your behavior correctly. Don't fool yourself. Once you've done that, then you can do something about the second mistake that keeps the rebellious self active.

Mistake # 2. Old Anger Is Not the Same as Current Anger

Once you recognize that you're not really asserting your independence by overeating, then you can ask yourself, What mistake am I making when I get so angry, and what can I do about it?

The problem is that old anger gets set off by fresh events in your contemporary life. The mistake you make is not being able to tell the difference, and because you can't tell the difference, the old situation and the current situation feel the same, and your defiant response seems like your only choice, just as it was when you were a child. If you can separate the two by stopping misinterpreting current events to mean the same as old events, then you can learn how to respond to the current situation and find the mature response that will make you truly independent.

Old anger was created and stored in our brains when as children we were disrespected, or not acknowledged or unappreciated, or misunderstood, belittled, controlled, or taken for granted. At the time this happened to you, you had only two major responses. You either displayed a furious temper or you seethed inside, too frightened to show what you really felt. In either case, if the anger was not resolved, you're still holding anger in some part of your brain, and you're extremely sensitive to any contemporary event that looks like or smells like or is in anyway similar to your particular sore spots (being belittled, unappreciated, taken for granted). You're primed to overreact, and primed to misinterpret.

My patient Janice was consumed with anger because of the special attention her older sister received from her mother. By age seven she had learned her lesson well. Any expression of anger about that subject brought only more coldness and scorn from her mother, and another victory for her sister. That's when she started to become fat, and an army of pediatric fat doctors couldn't do a thing about it. She remembers going down to buy boxes of candy in the same office building right after her weekly weigh-in as an adolescent.

As we traced her eating patterns as an adult, the most powerful trigger to her defiant eating occurred when she saw another woman, a slimmer and easier-to-be-with woman than she, get noticed and get the attention and care from the managers in her office. It was an easy and obvious "a-ha."

Eventually she learned to make the distinction between the normal office politics and what went on in her early family life. When she did that, and also acknowledged that she was being a little too angry and aggressive around the office and not so easy to like, she began to change her behavior, and her angry eating stopped.

Misinterpreting a present situation to mean the same as a past unresolved situation is everyone's weak spot, but just because something is normal behavior doesn't excuse us from the responsibility of being alert to this weakness, and trying to catch ourselves before we damage ourselves by overeating or damage someone else by projecting on them a degree of anger that they don't deserve. In Janice's office incident, she actually liked the woman who got all the attention and didn't want to go off on her, so eating aggressively to punish herself was the only way she found to deal with that anger.

Janice's solution to her anger eating represents one end of the spectrum. When she separated past sore spots from current reality, she understood that she had nothing to be angry about in the present. Nobody did anything unfair to her. She simply confused past and present, and the only action required by her was to look at her general attitude at work and make some changes for the better. That was her route to true independence, making defiant eating unnecessary.

But more often the confusion of past and present is really based on more subtle differences of degree. You are being insulted or misunderstood or disrespected by someone, and you are overly sensitive to it because of old anger. It's during those times that you have to rely on the principle that we have repeated many times in this book. Look to the reality of the situation, and start by assuming that all realities are complex and open to multiple interpretations. You have to be a "reality detective" and analyze each clue, and only after that decide on a response. You have to accept that your first blush of anger is a reflex based largely on a misinterpretation that the old anger situation and the current anger situation are the same. That needs to be followed by a thinking pause so you can see the difference.

There are many appropriate gradations of anger to be expressed in the real world that are dependent first on an accurate analysis of what is going on. Anger can be converted into energy for repair or progress (I was misunderstood, but I will show them) rather than expressed in a temper tantrum. Misunderstandings can be cleared up, compromises made, admissions of responsibility made. You might find that the insult that made you angry was unintentional or that you misunderstood, at which point your anger dissolves after the first exploratory conversation about what that was all about. You might decide that the insult was really born out of envy and competition, and in that way was really a compliment rather than a put-down. You might discover that your own entitlement and unrealistic expectations set up the disappointment, and there's no one to be angry at. These are just a few examples of what might be found out if the anger is analyzed and explored through several rounds of thinking through. Each "diagnosis" leads to a different action "cure."

True independence comes from acting appropriately, wisely, and maturely according to your own values of what is right and wrong. The more you keep your anger response keyed to the specifics of a particular reality situation, the more powerful you will be as a person. That will eliminate your defiant eating patterns.

You'll have to shrink yourself to fully recognize your real power, and that is where the exercises in part two will help you. You can also get some real help from the next chapter on emptiness, because at the bottom of emptiness is part of the answer as to why you haven't yet finished your autonomy maturation.

SHRINK YOURSELF SESSION NOTES
Develop a Mature Way to Deal with Anger

- You've learned that you're afraid of your own anger, so you eat to control it.

- You've learned that when you eat to deal with anger, you're attacking yourself rather than anyone else.

- You've recognized that eating to defy or punish someone only gives you a false feeling of power, and that's not real independence.

- You've learned the six different ways that you mask or excuse using food and fat as an aggressive weapon.

- You're beginning to see that you can recover your power by becoming more skilled at expressing anger appropriately in the context of very specific situations.

- You'll have to remember that you have two methods to void your powerless conclusion about anger and eating:
    1. Remember that rebellion and defiance are not the same as healthy independence and autonomy.
    2. Stop adding to your anger by confusing old anger with current situations.

8

Your Emptiness Layer

Our greatest pretenses are built up not to hide the evil and
the ugly in us, but our emptiness. The hardest thing to
hide is something that's not there.—*Eric Hoffer*

Ann, a forty-six-year-old married patient of mine who weighs 210
pounds, said, "I couldn't even begin to number the times I have
eaten to the point of being painfully full, but felt completely hollow
inside."

Feeling empty is both a psychological and a biological description. The biological reference is straightforward: my stomach cavity
is empty, my stomach is growling, I'm starved, and I must eat something to fill up. We all recognize that. The psychological description
starts out the same: I feel empty. But where that emptiness is actually located is unclear. Empty of what, and where is it? We get some
clue from those who are in mourning. They universally describe an
emptiness in the immediate aftermath of the death of a loved one
like I did when my parents and brother died. Sometimes they say,
"The world feels empty," but just as often they say, "I feel empty

inside, like something inside me has died," which it has, that is, their interior mind space and the existence of the person who has died is being reordered. Their relationship to the deceased, as represented in the images inside their mind, is being reorganized. The fullness that that person provided while alive is being emptied out.

There are many other times than mourning in everyone's life when we feel empty. People feel empty when relationships aren't working, or when their life is going in the wrong direction, or when they're too alone or unfulfilled, or even in a crowded room with loved ones.

Emptiness is the final layer of powerlessness we need to explore to relieve you of your phantom hunger. On the one hand, it's the easiest one to understand in relation to emotional eating. You feel emotionally empty, you conclude you're powerless, you eat, and for a few moments you feel full. There's a real feeling of fullness, but unfortunately it's not the fullness you're deeply longing for. There isn't a simpler explanation of emotional eating. But as is quite clear by now, we aren't focusing on the obvious, we're looking for the pause, the space between when you have the feeling of emptiness and then conclude that you're powerless to do anything about it, and how that experience of powerlessness is almost instantly transformed into the uncontrollable urge to eat.

On the other hand, the emptiness experience is intimately related to our most primal fear, the fear of abandonment, and that's very old and very complicated. Emptiness itself represents an absence, the absence of the nurturers who aren't there to pour love into that space. When we feel empty, we feel short on love. We've made this point in the Introduction and many times along the way: eating and filling up on food is a way to get love inside you. So now the thinking is ever more obvious. When I feel empty I'm in a state of love deprivation and powerless to do anything about it, so I get love from food. Food is my substitute love object, and when I eat I am reunited with that love object, and hope to be filled up with love. Of course, this cure is a myth, even though at times it feels so real, as we described in the food trance. But like all myths, they don't work in daylight. As you can see from Sally's statement below, food will never provide the love that she is really longing for.

The Futile Search for
Unconditional Love

An online member, Sally, who's sixty-eight, and two hundred pounds overweight, said, "The emptiness always seems to me to be about not being loved for who I am. Unconditional love. Something I didn't experience as a child; nothing I did was ever good enough for my parents. If I could unlearn the guilt, and begin to learn to love myself unconditionally, maybe I'd be able to stop the food addiction. As a child I snuck food into my room to cope with the physical and emotional abuse; it was my source of comfort."

The brain records experiences and wishes in images, not in words. The imagery of this myth, of being reunited with the perfect unconditional love object who gives, understands, accepts, encourages, guides, and adores us, is the same bedrock image that drives all of us to have and keep and work on our intimate relationships. We're always working toward, but never reaching, that goal of having a perfect source of love in adult life. Unconditional love is a rare and short-lived experience usually found only briefly and intermittently, in the parent–child relationship. When relationships fail to provide us with that feeling of unconditional love we so desperately crave, as they always will, then we go looking for it somewhere else. For some it's in alcohol, for others it's in sex, and for you, if you're reading this book, it's probably in food.

We insist on getting from somewhere or someone the unconditional love we're certainly entitled to have. The problem is that the sense of entitlement and reality clash. We're left in a stubborn and self-defeating position of insisting, waiting, and always being disappointed. In this area of our life, we live in denial.

Emptiness Is Part of All the Other
Layers of Powerlessness

I asked several hundred people struggling with weight control to tell me what it meant to them when they felt empty and compelled to overeat. They all started with the awareness that emptiness triggered their uncontrollable urge to eat but also that food didn't satisfy their emptiness for very long. Just as my patient Ann said above, the hollowness was still there no matter how much she put in her stomach. Filling up but still on empty was the universal experience.

"I eat when my husband goes away on business trips." Or, "I feel an aching emptiness inside that only food seems to fill, but only briefly," or, "I eat and eat and still feel like you could hear echoes inside me," and finally, "I chew so I don't have to hear the quiet."

When emptiness points to another layer of powerlessness, you're well on your way to being able to understand and master it.

How You Can Fill All That Emptiness

Emptiness is a normal human emotion, uncomfortable yet normal. Finding passions, diversions, and things to focus your efforts on can quell the normal occasional emptiness that we human beings are bound to feel. There are many real ways to fill that emptiness besides eating. You'll see how the experience of emptiness fits into one of the other four layers of powerlessness that we've already covered in *Shrink Yourself*.

Emptiness and the Self-Doubt Layer of Powerlessness

Theresa has struggled with her weight her whole life. She's a fifty-three-year-old college student who went back to get her degree after her children left home. She's had fifty-pound shifts in weight her whole life. When discussing emptiness with her I asked, "Is something missing?" She said, "Yes, there is. Love. Self-love. Acceptance. Self-acceptance. Tolerance. Self-tolerance. Forgiveness. Self-forgiveness. Respect. Self-respect. Like my mother was with me, I'm critical and demanding of myself, so I never feel good enough or worthy." You can see that her emptiness comes from the self-doubt layer. To address it, she'll have to do the self-doubt exercises in part two.

Emptiness and the Frustration/Reward Layer of Powerlessness

The following two people describe how the emptiness relates to the reward/frustration layer of powerlessness. They have some area in their life where they feel defeated, they've stopped pursuing their dreams, they haven't lived their potential, and without the real rewards that fulfillment gives, they can only give themselves the reward of eating.

George is a forty-six-year-old man who's preparing to have lap band surgery. He weighs 380 pounds. He said, "I think the emptiness is the 'what ifs' in life. What if I had gone to college, joined the army, learned to swim. I've spent my whole life being afraid to live. I spent a lot of time wondering why and wanting to change things but being too afraid to try. I guess the food trance is the moment I can forget the 'what ifs' and be in that moment only. The food trance is my temporary fix."

Peg is a thirty-six-year-old mother of four. She weighs 210 pounds. "I think for me, the emptiness is feeling unfulfilled in life. I've always tested very high. I have an IQ in the genius range but I don't finish things. I guess maybe I'm looking for some kind of satisfaction. I sure have *finished* my share of pretzel bags, though."

These people will have to do the work in part two to determine what would really fulfill them in life.

Emptiness and the Safety Layer of Powerlessness

Aisha, an online member who's forty-five years old and weighs 175 pounds, said, "I never feel like I'm enough. I was raised by an extremely abusive mother. I barely remember the physical abuse, but the verbal/emotional abuse is still with me. I have a degree, I've raised two wonderful children, been married to the same man for over thirty years, held a top management job for eighteen years, and still I always feel like I'm hiding from my mother. I feel empty all the time, like I'm 'waiting' for life to start."

She'll have to work toward realizing that fat can't protect her from what happened to her years ago. She needs to create a real sense of safety inside herself so that she can make her life begin now.

Emptiness and the Rebellion Layer of Powerlessness

My patient Amelia, who is fifty-one and has been on diet after diet in her life, said, "As a small child, my parents decided to move from the city to the suburbs. I left my friends, my school, my home, and most importantly my grandparents, whom I would visit every day. The place that they moved me to was far away and our nearest neighbor was a quarter of a mile away, a very stark contrast to where I had been living. Due to the change in environment (snow, proximity, etc.), we were housebound for days at a time. My parents weren't getting along. My mother kind of checked out—sleeping all day, not really caring what her two small children were doing (I was six and my sister was four). So my sister and I ate and ate and ate. Whatever we wanted, however much we wanted. My dad was a police officer at the time and worked a very weird schedule. He would take care of us when he was home and in the absence of my beloved grandparents, this was all the supervision we received. Eating at that time was twofold: we ate out of boredom, we ate out of loneliness, we ate out of the sheer fact no one was watching, we ate to prove we could, we ate to fill the empty space of not having our friends or our grandparents around us anymore. This is when food started to become an issue."

As a child, Amelia used food to assert her independence and to fill the emptiness she felt. She has been trying to fill that emptiness with food ever since. Working on the rebellion layer of her experience of powerlessness helped fill in her emptiness.

The Mystery Layer of Emptiness

Underneath all of these other meanings of emptiness is the mystery layer of emptiness. What about that emptiness that's not about your life today, but your life so long ago that you couldn't possibly remember it? Is there anything you can do about that? Some of the descriptions of emptiness I received expose this layer.

Steve, a fifty-eight-year old man who is forty pounds overweight and is an online member, said, "I often feel empty. I've been able to recognize this feeling for many years in myself, even as a very young child. It often seems very physical . . . something that I need to fix. I do feel like something is missing. From the outside, it would look like I've got what I need. I'm married to a beautiful woman, I have a beautiful son, a decent job . . . but it's never enough. I'm miserable. I hate my job, I feel unloved, I feel alone. I feel very alone. I can feel alone in a crowded room. I can feel alone in my own living room surrounded by family. I wish I knew what the big thing was that has been missing but at this point in my journey, I really don't know what that is."

For Steve, there was nothing for him to face or take charge of; there was just this unending, inexplicable emptiness constantly inside him. He was waiting for something that never happened.

The powerlessness that occurs when you interpret who you are as being someone who's empty, who's missing some important ingredient in your makeup as a person, means that you believe you have a hole in your psyche. That's an ancient image of infantile panic. It doesn't represent the reality of who you are.

Unfulfilled Expectancy

As you mature, you have to accept the fact that expectations often lead to disappointments and to gratification that is often delayed. That hurts, but it's tolerable. As infants and children, we expected our needs to be fulfilled and we expected them to be fulfilled quickly, or else we began to form catastrophe predictions. When infants have the image or feeling of not getting needs met, either the emptiness of their stomach or the emptiness of being alone, it makes them wail violently because their survival depends on it. But in a sense it's an early version of panic based on a catastrophe pre-diction. For the infant, it feels as if they'll never be fed or nurtured again, and this induces panic.

Delores, one of my online members, gives us a clue as to what this is like when she writes the following: "I really feel that a large part of my compulsive overeating stems back to when I was an infant. When I was a baby, I had a lot of allergies and when I was fed, I would immediately vomit my food up. It took a long time to get the right formula. My mother decided that it was not wise to feed a child who had just gotten sick to their stomach, so she didn't give me more food for another four hours. Then the same cycle would be repeated. Finally, my mother went back to work and a caretaker took over and told my mother she couldn't fill me up, that I was starving. I often think that I have a deep-seated psychological urge to con-tinue eating even when I'm not hungry because I don't know when I'm going to get food again. I know that this isn't rational. I'm an adult and control my food sources. But it's almost like I *have* to have the food available or I feel like I'm going crazy, and then of course when it's available, I eat it. How can I overcome this emotional need? I can't go back and change being that infant or the circum-stances surrounding my early years, but there has to be a way to overcome the insatiable psychological need for food."

What Delores is experiencing is not irrational, it's biological. Her latent sense memory (located in her brain cells) of panic, based on a catastrophe prediction of absence (abandonment), is being acti-vated. The way you remedy the problem is the same no matter when it started. You'll need to prove to yourself, one food choice at a time, that you won't go crazy the way your expectancy pattern predicts. Going crazy is a catastrophe prediction. The image in her mind is that if she doesn't have food immediately at hand, that absence will drive her crazy. That image is entirely at odds with reality. Assuming that she's a well-functioning adult with the ability to go to the grocery store and pay for food, then food is no more than a few min-utes away. Her image is a memory of unfulfilled expectancy. In her mind, she believes that if she doesn't get the food immediately, she may never get it. That's the empty hole in her psyche. It's a bodily memory summarized in that image. The story about her first years was obviously told to her and helps her explain what she's now remembering and feeling, but even without that history, we could read in her current behavior that she has a level of expectancy and fear of abandonment that hasn't evolved over the years, and is the root cause of her unrelenting hunger.

Expectancy Extends beyond Food

Not everybody has an allergic eating experience in infancy, but everyone does have a feeding experience of some kind, and an ongoing relationship with the same parents who continue to feed you different kinds of love than food throughout your life. Depending on how that relationship forms and is transformed over the years, you'll be imprinted with some kind of expectancy of love and nurturance that will organize your whole style of relating to others, especially intimates and family members. What I'm about to describe is an almost universal experience in the patients I see for weight problems, but may not be your exact experience.

When you experience emptiness in everyday life, it becomes a threat to whoever now represents the love your parents did or didn't give, because you're on the hunt for unconditional love, and are bound to be frustrated. More specifically, the threat that exists inside you when you're "empty" is based on the catastrophe prediction that nobody is going to be there for you in your time of need. You'll be powerless in a way that only a totally helpless infant can be powerless, and that's an unbearable feeling. When the experience of emptiness strikes, you're flooded with feelings that nobody really cares, that you're not even in their thoughts. You can't count on anyone to soothe or nurture you, and you can't do it for yourself. You're alone, floating in some alien, empty, cold space, without a tether to the familiar or the reliable. That's the hollow, empty experience.

What keeps this emptiness alive is not what happened in your infancy, though; it's what keeps on happening because of the conclusion that you've come to. That conclusion is that you cannot trust anybody to really be there for you, so you can't let anybody really fill you up with the warmth of a human relationship. You keep yourself empty in the following way.

When your abandonment fear is activated, you have such a fear of rejection and disappointment that you pull back when a deep trust and fondness is growing with someone. You start to get filled with something, get afraid, and so empty yourself of what's being given to you. You're so afraid of abandonment that even when someone is offering real love and nurturance, you perceive it as something that can't be trusted. Whatever is being given is seen as temporary, tantalizingly dangerous, certainly not going to last, and more than likely a manipulation of some sort. You freeze, shut down, empty out: that's how you protect yourself.

Because the route to real filling up by accepting the love that's there for you is closed down by your fears and mistrust, you turn to food. You have fulfilled your prophecy that no one will be there for you by not letting them be there for you, so you're powerless to get the love you want, and you must eat.

When you feel this way, food becomes the cure. If you fill up, you banish the threat of abandonment that the emptiness represents because in those moments of fullness you're reconnected. You've prevented the predicted abandonment. When food reconnects you in this way, it represents the unconditional love of a perfect mother. It's more reliable than any human mother (or husband or wife or lover) could possibly be. It's always there. It'll never abandon you, whereas human mothers and spouses do terrible things like die, or have lives of their own, or turn their attention to others, or are self-obsessed, or are emotionally illiterate, or are barely holding on themselves, or have to work, or don't protect you.

The Way Out of Emptiness

Whenever you overeat in response to the kind of emptiness experience I have just described, you are tacitly agreeing that you aren't an adult, but are still a helpless infant in fear of abandonment. It's not the truth, but it's a version of the truth that you keep alive this way. As you learned in the very beginning of this book, it's a universal experience that on some unconscious level, childhood fears of abandonment get reduced to one almost palpable image of an empty cavity that can be filled only by something outside, as if we're still infants with open mouths waiting for milk, screeching like the baby birds being fed in nature films. That primal, early memory of being hungry—of being voracious and unattended to, desperately needing milk in order to survive and feel comforted and loved, in order to avoid discomfort—gets implanted in our psyches, and we recall it as a potential disaster state. We fear that maybe no one will be there to fill that void, and then it'll go on endlessly, while we helplessly wait in anguish.

The familiar empty feeling that any emotional eater can tell you about is only an inch away from abandonment terror. As long as you believe that such terror is too horrible to experience, the food trance will have a seductive power over you.

The cure for this is based on a cliché. Remember, that was then, this is now.

SHRINK YOURSELF SESSION NOTES
Finding Real Fulfillment

- You'll have to reinterpret the experience of emptiness to see exactly what it means to you and how you can take charge of your life to deal with it.

- You'll have to catch yourself in the mystery layer of emptiness. You'll have to recognize, not avoid, your abandonment fear, and see it for what it is, an outdated image and memory of what you feared as a child.

- You'll have to become intimately acquainted with your expectancy pattern and the catastrophe prediction you make about being deprived or disappointed.

- You'll have to prove to yourself, by the experience of catching yourself, that your expectancy pattern is not the right way to deal with your relationships in life.

- You'll have to stop adding to your emptiness by mistrusting what is being given to you by those who love you.

- You'll have to remember that you have two methods to void your powerless conclusion about emptiness:

  1. Remember that emptiness can never be filled with food.

  2. Stop adding to your feelings of emptiness by confusing your childhood fear of abandonment with the current situation.

PART TWO

The Practice Sessions

9

Recovering Your Power

> The way to recover the meaning of life and the
> worthwhileness of life is to recover the power
> of experience. This can be done.—*Abraham Maslow*

When you started reading this book, you thought you were here to simply look at your feelings of powerlessness over your uncontrollable urge to eat. What you've been discovering is that that top layer is just a cover-up for the five other layers of powerlessness. The five types of power that you'll need to recover are:

1. Power over your self-doubts.
2. Power over how you deal with frustration and get rewarded in life.
3. Power to create your own sense of safety.
4. Power to deal with anger without rebelling.
5. Power to fill your own feelings of emptiness.

Countless patients have proved to me that once you can recover your power in those other areas, recovering your power over the uncontrollable urge to eat becomes almost effortless. This is what I've been talking to you about for the whole book so far. How to remedy the problem probably feels like the farthest thing from a magical solution to weight loss that you could ever imagine. But there's more at stake here than your weight, as important as your weight is. It's been my observation and experience that using weight to manage the emotions and circumstances in your life does far more damage than merely giving you a body you're dissatisfied with; it keeps your whole life functioning in a less than optimal way. Managing your weight and managing your life are so intricately interwoven that there can't be a simple solution. It's never simple to manage your life. I would not be pointing these things out to you unless I knew unequivocally that you can in fact recover your power over food and your whole life if you're willing to do the work.

Simplifying *Shrink Yourself*

Let's review everything you've learned so far in the most simple terms I can think of. This will set the stage for sessions that follow, where you start to acquire the observational experiences that lead to change.

If you're an emotional eater, then up until now this is how you've dealt with life: Something happened (an event or interaction); you felt powerless in one of the five ways we've talked about; and, in an effort to alleviate the pain of that powerlessness, you overate and then regretted it.

In part two, in order to recover your power, I show you how to change that pattern into something that looks more like this: something happens (an event or interaction); you feel powerless in one of the five ways (which you'll now be able to observe, recognize, and identify); you'll feel the panic of that powerlessness come on but you'll be able to pause and analyze what you're feeling. You'll compare your inner reality (your self-doubts, your fears, your past experiences) to what is actually happening (your external reality), and you'll respond to what is happening in your current reality and find that you no longer have the uncontrollable urge to eat.

All the things you'll learn to do in part two teach you how to convert the experience of powerlessness to powerfulness. Each time you can effectively deal with your experience of powerlessness without short-circuiting feelings with food, you'll become a more mature and ultimately a more efficient person. You'll have to prove this to yourself—one experience at a time, one food choice at a time—until who you are and how you deal with life are different. It won't happen all at once. Remember that you've reinforced your powerlessness for years every time you chose to eat instead of tackling what was really bothering you. It will take time to unravel, but it can be done. In fact, every person who has achieved lifelong weight loss and given up their obsession with food has *learned* to do it.

You'll have to stop adding to your existing feelings of powerlessness by misinterpreting the events in your life. The events that you'll have to watch out for are the following:

- Anytime you measure yourself or feel that you're being measured.

- Anytime you don't know how to handle frustration and you think that food is the only reward you can get.

- Anytime you don't feel safe.

- Anytime you feel angry but don't know how to deal with the anger.

- Anytime you feel empty.

Once you can stop immediately misinterpreting these kinds of experiences in a way that leaves you feeling powerless, you'll start to discover other options besides eating. You don't have to do this on your own. I'm going to show you how.

The *Shrink Yourself* Method

At this point in the book, I expect and hope, that you have the following dilemma. "On the one hand, I now understand how emotional eating works, and along the way I've had some good insights about myself and my experiences of powerlessness, and have some idea about what I can do about it. On the other hand, it seems overwhelmingly complex and I don't have much confidence that I can actually change my behavior in a way that can be sustained." If that's your dilemma, let me assure you that you're just where you should be. No one can simply transform all that you've read into new behavior.

That's what the next part of the book is designed to do, to help you change, by a slow and steady integration of new learning based on new experiences. What I want to help you achieve is a naturalistic, not a forced self-conscious, change. The goal is to find yourself changed without quite knowing why it happened. One online member said: "By week five of the program, I was amazed at how much insight I had gained, and how easy it was to make good food choices."

I want to keep your conscious mind active to give your unconscious mind what it needs to do the work of integration. By now you know a lot about emotional eating: you know what it is, how it starts, and what keeps it going. But what you don't know yet is how to stop it. In this next part of the book, the practice sessions, I'll help you apply what you learned in part one to overcome emotional eating once and for all. By the end, you'll know exactly what to do when you feel powerless over food or powerless in your life.

Having the right information doesn't necessarily lead to smart food choices, although it's always a good start. For real change to happen, especially change involving your eating habits, you need to arrive at a series of personal insights about your life and about how you process your experiences and emotions. The insights I'm referring to are the ones that make behavior change natural. Alcoholics sometimes refer to them as "moments of clarity." The insights you should strive for are the ones that help you realize you're not powerless over food—insights that help you realize there are better, easier, and healthier ways to deal with your problems than seeking the escape that food has provided up until now.

When I work directly with patients, I help the insights that lead to behavior change arrive more quickly then if my patients were on their own. However, I must accept that I can't force the insights on them. I may know exactly what a particular patient must realize before they can feel better, but I can't force them to see it my way, or to see it when I see it.

The insights must come from inside the patient when they're ready. It's the same with you. In the sessions that follow, I'll give you exercises designed to help gather important insights, but you have to do the exercises and make the observations. You can learn only by having new experiences that I hope to create for you in each exercise. Just reading through the text might help a little, but it's up to you to do the work. You must make it your own.

As we continue together, pretend you're a patient or a member of my Shrink Yourself online course. Each chapter that follows will be like a session with me. You'll do a series of exercises and read stories that'll help you to understand why the exercise is important. As you go along, each session will build on the sessions that come before.

This "progressive disclosure" parallels what happens in therapy. During traditional therapy, the patient and I can examine deeper issues in each new session only because we know more than we did in the previous session. One memory or thought or observation triggers another, and the web of thoughts and feelings that compose the conscious mind comes alive in a new way. I've tried to make this happen for you in the sessions that follow by sequencing the exercises so that each simple piece of awareness is linked to other insights until you see things from a perspective that you didn't have before. You'll actually go through a series of transformations having the exact experiences in the right sequence that you need to transform the way you manage your weight and your life.

Let's start with an anecdote now, to put you in the mood for the work ahead. One of my patients, Helene, told me that she faces a desperate, losing battle every time she sits down to eat—chocolate cake versus carrots, calories versus willpower. She calculated that if she lived to be seventy-nine years old—the average life expectancy for an American woman—she would have to make the right dietary choices approximately 80,000 times! In other words, she faced

80,000 future struggles—a horrifying prospect, and yet a prospect that most overweight people face. Helene had already tried several major diets without success. She had no idea how to comfort herself without resorting to food. I'm assuming that like Helene, you want to avoid 80,000 future struggles. So come into my office and have a seat.

The sessions that follow will help you to find that mature, powerful part of yourself, and to do something about your long-term struggle so you can win the weight war.

By the time you finish the last session, you'll have a plan in place for making wise eating choices no matter what emotions you're facing or what types of crises you're enduring or how good or how bad your luck is tomorrow. You may still, on occasion, want to avoid confrontation, or chase away a bad mood with food, but most of the time you'll know better, and have good alternative options.

You'll find that having a blank notebook will help you to do the work in the sessions that follow. So find a notebook and let's get started! If you prefer, check out the online step-by-step companion program to this book at shrinkyourself.com and do the program while reading the book.

10

SESSION 1
Getting Started

People say that motivation doesn't last. Well, neither does bathing—that's why we recommend it daily.—*Zig Ziglar*

In this session:

- You'll define yourself as an emotional eater.
- You'll look at the differences between phantom hunger and physical hunger.
- You'll have to remember that in the gap between powerlessness and the uncontrollable urge to eat, you're making a decision that can be changed. You'll start to observe that gap, so you do indeed have a choice.
- You'll have to rid yourself of denial in order to do the learning work that will free you from your food addiction by looking at your misguided motivations to lose weight and at your failure strategies.

Now you have to decide whether you really are ready to do the work necessary to master your emotional eating patterns, or you are just here to "think about" it some more. It's easy to deceive yourself about this issue. If you're here to get it done, I can help you do that. If you're here to think about it, the best I can do is help you think about thinking about it, and maybe you'll decide to be serious about doing something, or maybe you just aren't ready.

By now you know that weight is an emotional issue. Believe me—resistance is common when it comes to weight loss, and chances are good that you harbor some yourself. Some people get so agitated when discussing weight issues that they can't focus on logic. They feel that nobody understands how hard they've tried to diet or what it feels like to be unable to lose weight—that they've been subjected to bad advice for years and years. If you fit this category, you certainly might find yourself resistant to the ideas that you've learned about in this book. And so, before we continue with the exercises, we need to sidestep a bit to address your mind-set and to look at any ways you might have of deceiving yourself into thinking you've been doing work that you actually haven't started. If you're 100 percent sure that you don't suffer from one bit of ambivalence or self-deception or resistance regarding weight loss or life change, you can skip this session. Otherwise, please read on.

There's a principle of psychotherapy that I want to apply here. My patients always start out ambivalent. They want relief from their problems and know that they'll have to make some changes, but they fear making those changes because altering old patterns is difficult.

We therapists know this, so we expect ambivalence, meaning that although we know you'll want to change, we also recognize that you'll resist making those changes. In therapy, we work with the ambivalence. It's expected, it's real, and it makes sense that it would manifest as you read this book.

Your Resistance Decoded

It came as a surprise to me when during my first public lectures on emotional eating, some audience members became hostile. Most nodded and were eager to find out what they could do about their relationship to food, but a few people thought I was accusing them of something. (Of course, I should've been smarter about this and remembered the very same principle of resistance that I'm outlining here, but I wasn't.)

One woman in the audience explained that she'd been a heavy child, and ever since grade school, she'd been accused of choosing to be fat, of being weak-willed, stubborn, and lacking in willpower. No one understood her agonizing conflict, and she was tired of being preached to and pushed to change. She'd misunderstood my message, taking it as yet another accusation, until I assured her that I agreed with her assessment that lack of willpower wasn't the culprit. Others in the audience took great objection to the psychological approach, feeling that I had implied they were somehow defective, and they didn't want any such labels cast at them. It quickly became clear to me that I'd entered a minefield filled with anger, despair, and hurt. These people felt victimized by a myth perpetuated by the diet industry—a myth asserting that people stay fat because they don't have enough self-discipline.

"We have as much willpower as our skinny neighbors," one audience member told me, and I agreed. There are many overweight people who are highly disciplined exercisers and demonstrate as much discipline as anybody else at work and at home. It's not a trait we're talking about, it's an area of unresolved conflict. I recognized the understandable outrage she felt. And yet I noticed something else, something that concerned me because I saw how it could sabotage any sincere dieting effort. I saw denial—the same type of denial that sabotages people trying to kick any harmful addiction. Those agitated audience members had experienced so much misunderstanding, so much pain and denigration around their weight issues, that they no longer could face reality. They'd slammed the door on themselves and didn't want to consider that their weight problem had anything to do with their life, preferring any other cause than that. They didn't want any more probing or self-exploration into the sore spots of their psyche; it was off-base, and all the evidence to the contrary had to be denied.

If you feel like one of those angry audience members, please understand—the *Shrink Yourself* method does *not* allege that you have a sickness or a disease. Instead, *Shrink Yourself* says that you have an agonizing conflict within yourself because, for one reason or another, food has become implanted in your mind as a mood control mechanism and you haven't yet proven to yourself that you can regulate your life without the use of this mechanism. That's the prime reason you've been afraid to do the exploration of yourself that you need to succeed. You've already prejudged yourself and determined that you won't survive emotionally intact if you don't use food as a tranquilizer anymore. You happen to be wrong, but you won't be able to believe what I'm telling you until you've finished the book and discover that for yourself. I'm here to coach you in your battle with yourself, to help you explore that painful conflict within, to help you find a healthy way to resolve your internal discomfort. I understand how scary it can be to investigate what lies below the surface, but it's better to be a little scared of the journey than to close the door. I promise that we'll proceed through the exercises slowly and carefully, step by step. I simply ask for your willingness to give it a try.

Let's start with the biggest stumbling block most dieters trip over—the idea that willpower alone should win the weight war. Of course you have willpower—you wouldn't have ever attempted a diet if you didn't and you can't possibly function in life without it, but willpower alone isn't enough. Why not? Because the adversaries you face overpower willpower.

You know you have willpower, but maybe you think you don't have enough. That's a familiar self-accusation. "I'm lacking some vague but important ingredient. I just don't have enough, so why try again?" Aha . . . another form of denial, in this case the denial of self-efficacy. "I'm missing something, so I can't really be responsible for my failure. It's outside of my control." It all comes down to feeling helpless—powerless.

Sometimes overweight patients will tell me that they feel as if they're being controlled by some inner persona that overpowers them and always wins—a demonic other. This quote from a morbidly obese patient of mine illustrates this well. "There is a voice that says,

'Ellen, let's go to the Cheesecake Factory and let's have some of that cake, the one with the caramel on the top or maybe some cookies. Yes, chocolate chip cookies—the ones from the mall. That's right, we want cookies.' It's almost as if I have renters living in my body. I have at times, at the voice's insistence, gotten up in my pajamas, thrown on a top, and ran to a twenty-four-hour grocery and bought as much as eighty dollars' worth of treats."

I've no doubt that this experience is real. I've heard it described by hundreds of patients in my office, and thousands of people who've taken the Shrink Yourself program mention this adversary frequently. People addicted to food because of emotional eating feel powerless, want to and need to lose weight, but just can't do it or do it for very long because there's some other person inside them who takes over and sabotages their best intentions.

There's no demon inside, even though it feels like that. The reason I know this is a self-delusion is that so many people start this way and, through the process we're going to use, deconstruct the "demon," and it disappears. But if you believe in your demon and your powerlessness, you'll never have a chance to test whether what I'm saying here will be true for you, because you'll only be willing to put in a halfhearted effort, and that won't work.

So remember the next time you experience that "irresistible urge": you're just observing one or more of your powerful motivations to overeat, which is overriding your good judgment. And if you can't catch it in time to unmask it before you indulge, at least try to identify what it was after the fact. Creating a pause that's long enough for you to think before a binge is a huge first step. In that pause, you might be able to let your feelings tell you what they're really longing for and not eat at all, or at the very least you might be able to make a better food choice.

Reconfirming That You're an Emotional Eater

In part one, we defined emotional eating, and you saw to some degree how it functions in your life. However, it's very easy to backpedal and begin denying that you personally are struggling with emotional eating. Fortunately, there's a very easy way to decide whether you really are an emotional eater—we'll look at your symptoms.

Emotional Eating

All diagnoses start with observing symptoms. If you have a runny nose, itchy eyes, and can't stop sneezing, you conclude that you have a cold because you have the symptoms of one. We'll do the same for emotional eating.

Below is a list of questions, plus a few more, that we asked you at the beginning of the book. These questions cover the most common symptoms of emotional eating. If you answer yes to many of the questions, you have the symptoms of emotional eating, and you can therefore conclude that you are one.

1. Do you ever notice your hunger coming on fast?

2. When you get hungry, do you ever feel an almost desperate need to eat something right away?

3. When you eat or snack, do you often eat mindlessly, not paying attention to the taste of the food or how much you are eating?

4. When you get hungry, do you sometimes feel you need a certain type of food or treat to satisfy yourself?

5. Do you ever feel guilty after you eat?

6. Do you experience an urge to eat when you are emotionally upset?

7. Do you eat to get rid of a feeling of emptiness?

8. Do you stuff food in quickly, almost as if you were trying to stuff yourself?

9. Have you tried to lose weight before, only to find your efforts derailed by your urge to eat?

10. Do you ever feel powerless over your desire to eat unhealthy foods, or powerless to control your portions of healthy foods?

If you answered yes to three or more of the questions above, you're experiencing the symptoms of emotional eating, which means you're an emotional eater. As we move forward, keep in mind that these symptoms are not the real problem; rather, they're the indications of the real problem. It's time to make a decision: Are you an emotional eater? If yes, admit it! If no, give this book to someone who is.

EXERCISE

Ten Healthy Eating Habits You Should Adopt

You might still be thinking, *I have the symptoms but that doesn't mean I have to do anything about emotional eating. I can still control my weight by some other approach.*

If you didn't think you needed to do something about your emotional eating, you wouldn't even be reading this book. So this argument is at least partially wrong from the get-go. But it's wrong for another reason as well.

Because you're an emotional eater, you can't be a rational eater, and therefore you won't be able to control your weight. No other method will work. Below is a list of the ten healthy eating habits anyone who manages their weight must follow. Next to each of the ten eating habits there is an "I" statement. If you can say the statement out loud and feel as if you're telling the truth, then you know that habit is not a problem for you. If you feel like you're lying when you make the statement, write that one in your notebook so you can remember to work on it later.

Habit # 1: Listen to Your Body

I stop eating when I'm full and only eat when I am hungry.

Habit # 2: Manage Your Hunger

I feed myself properly through the day so I don't lose control.

Habit # 3: Bounce Back

If I've made a poor food choice, I don't use that as an excuse to eat everything in sight.

Habit # 4: Keep Your Weight in Mind

I keep my weight in mind when I make food choices.

Habit # 5: Avoid Junk Food

I mostly avoid junk food.

Habit # 6: Exercise Enough

I exercise enough to stay healthy.

Habit # 7: Control Your Portions

I know how to properly control the amount of food I eat.

Habit # 8: Prevent Binges

I know when I'm about to binge and can stop myself.

Habit # 9: Savor Your Food

I eat good food in a slow way so that I enjoy it.

Habit # 10: Choose a Balanced Diet

I make sure I eat a healthy, balanced diet that keeps me feeling good both physically and mentally.

If you're like most of my patients struggling with weight loss, you could only honestly say that you practice two or three of these habits. The reason that you don't practice the other simple habits is because of emotional eating.

Think about how much you want to lose weight, or how much you want to stop food from being the centerpiece of your life. Do you think that desire should be enough to control your portions, or avoid junk food, or practice any of those simple habits? It should be, but it's not. It's not enough because you're struggling with emotional eating. Trying to fully practice these habits is like trying to go to work with a temperature of 101. You might really want to make it so you don't have to use a sick day; you may even get through the door, but you won't last long.

And what happens if you can't practice these habits? Simple:

you gain weight, can't lose weight, or struggle to maintain your weight. It's as simple as that. Emotional eating leads to the inability to practice these habits, which leads to weight gain, which leads to you wanting to lose weight, which leads to you reading this book.

So when the part of you that wants to keep eating says you can happily live with the symptoms of emotional eating, or that those symptoms are no big deal, you can obviously contradict it.

EXERCISE

The Red Flag List

Watching these ten habits can help you identify when you're struggling with emotional eating. Take your notebook out, about halfway down the page make a heading that says "Good Habits," and list any of the ten habits you're struggling with. At the top of the page, make a heading that says "Symptoms" and write down the relevant symptoms you identified above.

We'll refer to this from now on as the red flag list. Whenever you experience these symptoms or have trouble practicing these habits, you'll know that emotions are dominating your eating behavior. That's the starting point. Instead of just automatically and blindly continuing to eat, stop for a moment to catch yourself in an emotional eating episode. Investigate what you're thinking and feeling when the cravings seem overpowering. The red flag list provides you with the opportunity to prove to yourself that you're an emotional eater through direct and immediate experience, not just because you answered a few questions in a book. This red flag exercise will get you into the experience that we will probe layer by layer. All you have to do now is get a hazy but solid view of what it is; then we will dissect the experience, and you'll really learn what is going on during those moments when the uncontrollable urge arises.

As you know, with passionate motivation you can accomplish practically anything. Determination has led people to climb Mount Everest, swim the English Channel, conquer the hearts of their enemies. You probably started your diets with a burning motivation, but lost it because your motivation rested on a hope to achieve something that weight loss alone can't accomplish. Let me explain.

My patient Laurie told me about the difficulty she experienced when she dieted and lost a hundred pounds several years before she came to see me. She told me that she kept herself going by thinking about how, once she reached her goal, she would sign up for a dating service. She intended to go out with many attractive guys and hoped to settle on one who made at least $150,000 a year.

While losing weight certainly made Laurie more attractive to men, finding love falls into a completely different category. Weight loss offers no guarantees in the love department, and if you hope to attain a goal that can't be achieved merely by losing weight, your diet can't succeed. So Laurie's willpower worked only until reality intervened and she did not find her dream lover. A year after losing all the weight, Laurie regained it, plus more. Unless you want to lose weight for your own health and well-being, plain and simple, your diet will probably fizzle faster than a balloon on a hot stove.

You can't make any deals with life. You can draw up the contract, but life won't sign it, so don't fool yourself. Being honest with yourself is the only way to kick the emotional eating habit.

Laurie's story demonstrates how people trip themselves up in spite of burning motivation. You can't succeed if you diet to please other people or for some transient goal, like to fit into a size 6 in time for your sister's wedding. You can't make a deal with life that if you lose weight your dreams and wishes will come true. Losing weight won't make you a rock star, won't make you rich, won't make the prom king kick himself for neglecting to ask you out twenty years ago. Motivations such as these inevitably lead you back to eating, because they depend on variables you can't control. And when you can't control the variables, your willpower crumbles.

A new shape and a new level of conscious confidence can add to your success in life, but the magical wish to be excused from the hard work of dealing with reality is a setup for a harsh disappointment, a familiar justification to soothe yourself with food. In other words, the will to succeed that kept you going dissipates because the success you wanted couldn't be achieved through dieting alone.

Your goals absolutely must be intrinsic and achievable, and only goals completely within your control fit into this category. Only these types of goals keep your commitment alive.

Let's take a closer look at how you can sabotage your diet by unwittingly setting unrealistic goals. Suppose, for example, you eat to assuage the pain you feel because your husband, Chester, ignores you. You enjoy a slice or two of tiramisu and forget about Chester for a while. The yummy treat transports you to a place of sensual satisfaction, and it kind of spaces you out so that Chester's rejection of you doesn't loom as large.

Later, though, you get depressed because you really do want to lose weight to look good for Chester, so that maybe he'll chase you around the house again, and you resolve to diet. That night, Chester insults you and you want to spite him. You don't want to do what he wants you to do, so you lose your motivation to diet and remember that you still have a slice of tiramisu in the fridge. And so the cycle continues. You have real motivation to diet, but the motivation depends on Chester, and you can't maintain your determination when Chester fails to act according to plan.

The truth is that your decision to lose weight can't ever involve another human being, because humans often act outside the plans we have for them. Your diet can't be motivated by a desire to satisfy a parent or partner or friend or child who just might find something else to criticize even after you drop those pounds.

Again, most of us launch into diets with unrealistic expectations that inevitably undermine our efforts to lose weight, because when we don't see the life-changing results we hoped for, we get discouraged and return to bingeing. Dieting leads to weight loss and improved health and vigor—period, the end. From any rational point of view, getting thin and healthy should be reason enough to forgo the french fries, but as you've already discovered, irrational forces tend to win the food wars. The work you'll do in this book will help you to finally make rational decisions about whether or not you really want to eat your way to oblivion, versus facing those emotional forces that remain unresolved and that lead you to eat beyond your own control.

Even after you do all this, the part of you that wants to hold onto emotional eating has one more trick. It's the most insidious trick of them all, and if I were a betting man, I would bet at least part of my savings that you're somehow falling victim to it, too. Almost everyone I have ever met falls into this trap.

The last trick that the denial part of you uses to keep you attached to emotional eating involves unrealistic expectations. It's natural to dream about what you can achieve. In fact, it's healthy. However, this troublesome part of you uses this healthy activity against you. Here's what happens.

The troublesome part of you that we're talking about asks you what you want to get by losing weight. It encourages you to dream big, too big. It gets you to expect great changes from losing weight (as if losing weight weren't good enough in itself). Then, when those unrealistic dreams don't come true, it says that all the work you did was for nothing—that you are better off eating whatever you want, since you're not getting these expectations met. Basically, this part of you sets you up for failure. Why? So it doesn't have to give up emotional eating and doesn't have to address real problems directly. Let's take a look at how this works for you.

Each item in the list below has built-in expectations that can backfire in the way I just described. Select the ones that apply to you. Be as honest as you can about your dreams and expectations. If you lie, you're not fooling anyone but yourself.

EXERCISE

Motivation

"I want to lose weight so I can _____."

    have better self-esteem

    make my career go more smoothly

    relieve some of my moodiness, depression, or anxiety

make some hard decisions about the course of my life

make my life feel as if it's going somewhere

have more day-to-day fun

better handle the ups and downs of life

feel less burdened by responsibilities

feel more independent

be less critical of myself

stop envying the life that others have

be more free of doubts and fears

start being more sexually active

feel more deserving of the good things I have in life

shed some of my shyness or discomfort around people

be happier and more content

How many dreams did you select? Most people select over half the list, sometimes more if I don't explain beforehand why they're selecting them. When weight loss doesn't bring these things, which it can't, you get disappointed, and have a very good excuse to go back to emotional eating.

Am I saying you shouldn't strive to fulfill these dreams? Absolutely not. I'm saying that weight loss alone can never bring these sorts of results. You need to take other steps as well. Just because you lose thirty or even fifty pounds does not mean you'll automatically drop those self-doubts you've been struggling with your whole life. Just because you're skinny doesn't mean you'll have more fun. And let me assure you, there are plenty of thin sex-starved people in the world as well. Weight loss is not a magic wand. It won't make these sorts of things happen. It might help, but that's all.

Make a declaration to yourself that you'll lose weight only for the direct and immediate benefit of being more healthy. You can be happy if it also helps you reach some other goal. Declare to yourself that you're not going to make a deal with life where you'll lose weight only if you get the payoff you're after.

Avoid the Failure Strategies

Because most dieters have at least some unrealistic and conflicted reasons for losing weight, they tend to fall prey to what I call "the failure strategies." Before you can learn new eating strategies that will lead you to weight loss for a lifetime, you need to understand why the approaches you've tried so far haven't worked. Once you see how you sabotage yourself with misguided motivation and misdirected strategies, you'll find it easier to let go of the doomed methods you've relied on until now.

If you want to avoid wasting any more of your time and energy on strategies bound to backfire, then you have to give up relying on methods like these. First, let's take a close look at the six most common failure strategies. See if you recognize yourself as you read about these methods. In fairness, observe that failure strategy #1 may have more to do with the diet industry than with any hidden agenda on your part.

Avoid Failure Strategy #1: Deprive and Gorge and Do It Again

The most common failure strategy relies on deprivation and discipline and nicely avoids dealing with the issues that drive eating dysfunction. Of course, everything you know about weight loss to this point in your life endorses the discipline/deprivation approach, so it might seem odd to you to disparage it now, to reject it as a doomed method. Ironically, the diet industry endorses this strategy with great gusto, but as you know by now, 99 percent of all diets ultimately fail. Please notice that I'm not telling you to eat with abandon or to give up exercise—not at all. I'm simply letting you know that these approaches won't work on their own.

You've seen the results of the grit-your-teeth-and-give-up-pastry approach. Perhaps neighbor John runs five miles a day and still has a potbelly. Sister Lara goes to Weight Watchers, drops twenty pounds, and then gains it all back when her boyfriend jilts her. Uncle Ron follows the Zone Diet, although recently you noticed Heath Bar wrappers in his briefcase. And you gave up the afternoon scone, only to blow it all out after work on Fridays (and Thursdays and Wednesdays, too).

Every single diet book and diet plan leads to the deprive-and-gorge approach, and so this is the most common strategy. As you know, when you diet, you deprive yourself of what you really want, applying willpower and discipline to keep yourself away from the fridge. It's a painful and difficult thing to do, and unfortunately, the method doesn't work for long because you really don't want to deprive yourself. Eventually, your emotional eating patterns kick in, and then the diet ends.

My patient Mary, a thirty-seven-year-old married mother of two, subscribes to this deprive-and-gorge approach. I asked her what it would be like if she finally succeeded in controlling her weight. She said, "I would be on top of the world. Last year I lost about sixty-five pounds and I was a totally different person. I could wear really cool clothes instead of the dreaded plus-size fashions. I didn't hate what I saw in the mirror—it was a stranger looking back at me, but one I admired. I was able to get off my blood pressure medication—but somehow I knew it was only temporary because of my lifelong battle with fat. It started with a donut—one donut—and then I started to eat three or four at a sitting. Especially when my boss got cranky, donuts were my salvation. Now once again, I hate to buy clothes, I'm back on medication, my knees ache, and I'm feeling tired and hopeless again."

Mary had strong motivation to change, but she depended on food as a source of comfort, and so whenever she encountered problems she overindulged in eating. When the air cleared, she regimented her food intake like a drill sergeant. Like Mary, you need to use a method more satisfying than deprivation, a method that dismantles your dependence on food in times of trouble rather than a method that leaves you even more hungry for satisfaction than you already are.

Make a Declaration. Be Honest: Where Are You Now?

1. I believe diets alone will no longer work for me, and I'm totally open to exploring my emotional eating patterns.

2. I'm not convinced about diets not working and I am reluctant to learn more about my emotional eating patterns.

Avoid Failure Strategy #2: Gorge and Run

Jason was thin when he was younger because he ran 4 miles each morning, rain or shine, to justify his enormous appetite. Food was the only thing that calmed his anxiety, but he compensated for overeating by exercising, and he did manage to stay trim. If he had a fight with his wife, he would stuff himself at dinner and then go out and jog another few miles. They didn't talk things through because he literally would run away, which only led to more arguments and more running.

Jason's plan worked until he fell off his bicycle and suffered a knee injury. The injury didn't heal properly, and Jason had to give up running. He did not, however, give up bingeing because his anxiety had increased now that he couldn't run away. He was stuck.

By the time Jason came to me for help two failed marriages later, he was fifty-five and grossly overweight. He no longer exercised at all, and he lived alone—with a plate of cookies near his bedside.

Like Jason, many people adopt exercise as a weight-control strategy. Instead of learning new eating habits, they exercise like crazy, stuffing themselves full and then compensating by hitting the gym. This "binge-and-jog" strategy fails over the course of a lifetime for most people.

First, in order to compensate for eating excess, you have to exercise so much that you increase the risk of injury, which poses special problems. Any time you need to stop exercising in order to heal, your weight balloons up quickly. I've seen patients in my practice who put on substantial weight after injuries and then couldn't lose it, though they had been trim athletes at one time—albeit athletes with a food addiction. Also, if you continue to eat unhealthy foods in excess, you weaken your immune system no matter how much you exercise, and so the risk of illness increases, illness makes exercise difficult, and anytime the routine slackens, the weight returns.

To lose weight for life, you need to conquer food addiction, not merely run around it.

Make a Declaration. Be Honest: Where Are You Now?

1. I believe that using exercise on a routine basis to compensate for overeating will no longer work for me.
2. I still want to be able to overeat and use exercise to compensate for it.

Avoid Failure Strategy #3: Gorge and Purge

Early in her marriage, Jan tried bulimia to stay thin. She would eat two dinners and the better part of a cake every evening. Friends marveled at her ability to stay thin. What they didn't see was what she did when she went into the bathroom. When Jan finished stuffing herself, she would find a private place and force herself to throw up. As soon as she was finished, she promised herself never to do it again, but the next time she found herself bingeing, she had to purge to make up for it. She hated herself for doing this. During dinner at a friend's home, she was planning her exit strategy, hoping to find a safe toilet where the sound wouldn't be heard. Her husband saw her red eyes when she came back to the table, and although he said nothing, his expression conveyed silent disgust. Fortunately, Jan came to see me before she did permanent damage to her body. After intensive work around her emotional eating issues, Jan finally beat her addiction.

Bulimia is a very dangerous strategy. People die from the electrolyte imbalance that happens with chronic purging, or they get serious dental problems, they have various forms of malnutrition and vitamin deficiency, and a secret life of agonizing shame. They appear to be thin, "together" people on the outside, but they feel like frauds on the inside.

Make a Declaration. Be Honest: Where Are You Now?

1. I believe that using purging to compensate for overeating will no longer work for me.
2. I still want to be able to overeat and purge to compensate for it.

Avoid Failure Strategy #4:
Look Good for the Camera

Angie is a chiropractor and competitive bodybuilder who works out five days a week. Despite all her knowledge about the importance of a healthy lifestyle and her motivation to be an example to her clients, Angie has a weight problem. By day, in public, she eats perfectly balanced low-calorie meals. But at one in the morning, Angie wakes up and starts bingeing.

Angie's emotional eating habit affects her moods, her health, even her career. When she has her bingeing under control, she's trim, happy, and successful. But when her midnight binges get the better of her, she becomes fat, miserable, embarrassed, and uncomfortable with her patients. She tries to stop her binges by reminding herself of her obligation to serve as a role model for her patients—by attempting to shame herself into abstinence—and while this approach works for her during the day, it has no power at night.

Obviously, Angie has strong motivation to get her weight under control, and she periodically succeeds in doing so, but then the cycle starts all over again. Angie has been locked in this struggle for two decades. The shame of failure doesn't work. Her unconscious won't cooperate. It wakes her up with the imperative to make up for all the deprivation and stress of the day, which includes the pressure of performing for and fooling her audience.

I've seen many variations of this strategy, including losing weight for a specific event such as an upcoming wedding or family reunion, or making a public declaration that you've started a diet, or buying clothes that fit only if you lose weight, or paying to join a support group that encourages success but rejects you if you fail.

There are many other ways to set yourself up to "have to" succeed, all of which lead to failure because the basic emotional eating problem is not addressed. Try as you may, you can't fool your own unconscious mind.

Make a Declaration. Be Honest: Where Are You Now?

1. I am ready to give up the belief that I can only do something if I do it to get applause from others. I am ready to take charge for myself.

2. I can't see controlling my weight just for myself.

Avoid Failure Strategy #5: Trick Your Metabolism

In our "get it done yesterday" culture, many seek a magic pill to dissolve cellulite, reverse weight gain, and make getting thin a breeze. All the pharmaceutical companies are looking for the big blockbuster solution that will control the hunger gland. The last "miracle pill" released on the market, Phen-Phen, ended up killing people, but the drug companies haven't given up, because the American public would much rather take pills that kill hunger than address the emotional source of the compulsion to overeat.

Phen-Phen wasn't the first weight-loss medication to endanger health. Dexedrine, an amphetamine, was commonly used for weight loss but has largely been discredited. Many people who started taking Dexedrine to lose weight ended up addicted, less hungry and less dependent on food, but more dependent on the drug. Unfortunately, as the bumper stickers say, "Speed Kills." Speed (amphetamine) increases your resting metabolic rate so that you burn more calories without having to exercise, stimulates a more rapid heart rate, and makes you sweat more. You stay up later and you have more energy to move around, but you can't use the method for long without physical damage. The speed category includes Ephedra, which is a major ingredient of many herbal appetite suppressants.

The same problems exist with thyroid supplements. If your thyroid is intact, taking more to speed yourself up will work for a while, but at a cost to your natural balance. And as long as you continue to eat too much, the method won't work and your health will suffer.

Make a Declaration. Be Honest: Where Are You Now?

1. I am ready to give up the belief that there will be a magical solution to my weight problem.

2. I still believe there is a simple solution, like a pill, that I have yet to find.

Avoid Failure Strategy #6: Play the Blame Game

Do you curse parental genes for giving you a slow metabolism? If so, you've fallen prey to the last of the failure methods—blaming the extra pounds on your metabolism. You might say that the blame game is more of a "failure attitude" than a failure strategy, but here the watchword is "failure." As long as you believe that genetics predispose you to being fat, you can tell yourself that your hunger is written "in the stars" and indulge your emotional eating habit whenever life gets difficult, doing nothing to change the underlying pattern.

I have seen so many patients who have made this claim, supporting it by telling me how diligent they have been about exercising and how careful they have been about their food intake. When I do a detailed inquiry about their exercise and eating habits, it turns out that they have simply been fooling themselves. One patient, Joe, was a real classic. He didn't bother to count the three beers at night or the daily trip to the ice cream store. Somehow those calories didn't count. My other patients also failed to count little things that added up, and almost all didn't exercise nearly enough to compensate for what they ate.

As long as you blame the extra pounds on a slow metabolism, you've fallen prey to another ruse—unless you've been diagnosed with hypothyroidism or take certain prescribed medications. Some medications *do* cause weight gain, either by changing your metabolic rate, making you retain fluids, or affecting how your body converts calories to energy versus storing calories as fat. That's a different story. But if you don't have hypothyroidism or prescription drugs to blame, then your metabolic rate is in the normal range and you need to gain control over your eating habits in order to lose weight.

If you can't quite accept the idea that you can't blame metabolism, look at the latest research showing that high-strung people stay thin not because of metabolism, but simply because they fidget more and move around more than you do and therefore burn more calories. The study showed that sedentary people sat 163 more minutes a day than fidgety people, who took 7,000 more steps and expended 350 more calories per day—a nonrigorous form of exercise, perhaps, but one that does contribute to weight loss. And so, again, metabolism can't be blamed.

The average person consumes 60 million calories during his or her lifetime. In order to stay at a steady weight you have to expend 60 million calories. That's the basic balance. If you make the slightest mistake in this balancing act, you immediately become overweight. For example, if you're an average man who needs 2,700 calories a day to remain at a steady weight but you take in 2,800 and expend only 2,700, you will gain 12 pounds every year.

An apple is about 100 calories. That's just an apple a day difference. In other words, it's very easy to be overweight.

Make a Declaration. Be Honest: Where Are You Now?

1. I am willing to accept that I have to deal with the psychological aspects of eating.

2. I'm still thinking and hoping that the reason I am overweight is outside me.

Look at your answers and reflect on what they mean. If you selected the first decision for all six failure strategies, you're open-minded and ready to learn about yourself. If you selected the second decision on all of the failure strategies, you're totally resistant to learning about yourself and may want to think about your resistance more before going any further. Perhaps you can come back to this in a month or two. If you have a mixture of both 1s and 2s, you may still be resistant to change. The more 1s you have, the more likely you will succeed.

Embrace Reality

Now you've seen that the six failure strategies don't work because they all attempt to stimulate weight loss while keeping the emotional eating option intact. You've also seen that denial doesn't work because emotional eating does, in fact, make you fat. When you follow one of the failure strategies, you make a hopeless bargain with yourself: "I will deprive myself for a while as long as I can go back to bingeing sometime. I will discipline myself to run as long as I can eat as much as I want when I am anxious. I will risk my health and harbor a shameful secret of purging as long as I can stuff myself at dinner. I will suffer public shame in order to overeat again. I will mess up my insides with speed and attack my hunger rather than attack the sources of emotional eating."

These strategies circumvent the reality of emotional eating. They keep the emotional eating habit alive in a rainy-day bank account in case you need it to cope with the next life stress. Unfortunately, you can't win as long as you hold the eating remedy in reserve for difficult times, because reality guarantees that you'll backslide under stress, throw off that delicate "calories in–calories out" balance, and put the pounds right back on.

If you want to control your weight for a lifetime, you need to attack and dismantle your emotional eating habit. There is no way around this. First you need to cultivate realistic motivations so that your diet doesn't fall apart. Then you need to follow a realistic strategy that gets to the roots of your addiction, as the *Shrink Yourself* sessions will help you to do. Once you have your addiction under control, you'll be able to practice the habits of people who stay thin for life. You'll eat rationally, which means you won't deprive yourself. You won't be hungry. You'll enjoy food. You'll have your weight under control because you will be eating to fill your biological stomach, not your phantom stomach. That's the goal I want to help you reach.

EXERCISE
Observe

For the next week, instead of focusing on your diet, just focus on finding a pause right before you're about to overeat. Ask yourself what you're feeling. Did something bother you? Where are you when it happens? What time of day is it, and who are you with at the time? The more information you can gather about what happens for you right before you overeat, the better you'll be able to do the exercises that are to come.

So You're Really Ready to Lose Weight

For anyone who has ever been in a bad relationship—and that's most of us—you know how hard it is to end the cycle. Your relationship with food is no different. You think you'll be too alone and empty without it and that you won't be able to function, but you're wrong.

You've accumulated a lot of good reasons why you don't want to give up your eating pattern. The smart thing to do is to no longer deny that you're hesitant or afraid to give up this pattern. Once you do that, you might be able to begin resolving the issue and shrinking yourself. Try it, and see if it works for you.

But to do that, you have to think things through, and therein lies the conflict that we'll start to address in this practical part of the book. You've probably used food to avoid thinking things through so many times that you no longer have the confidence that you can face your feelings and end up better off.

When you don't go deeply into your feelings, you can only think about the issues on a superficial and unproductive level and that keeps you stuck, which is the all-too-familiar cause of phantom hunger. When you no longer use food to stop your feelings, you'll not only stop being a slave to food, but you will begin to have mastery over many areas of your life. If you agree that you're ready to *Shrink Yourself*, let's dig in.

11

SESSION 2
Conquering the Feeling Phobia

In the next two sessions:

- You'll identify your feeling phobia.

- You'll start to develop the skills to understand what you make your feelings mean, how you misinterpret things, how you form catastrophe predictions, and what your powerlessness conclusions are.

- You'll identify the benefits of being in the food trance, the escape it gives you, and the pleasure it provides.

- You'll examine what it costs you to retreat into the food trance instead of facing your feelings, especially the fact that it keeps you from solving the problems that need to be solved.

- You'll identify the other ways you can get a time-out when feelings become too intense.

- You'll learn to master the feeling phobia and food trance, and then you'll be ready to understand the deeper issues that make you feel powerless.

In the first session I helped you with a series of exercises so that you could begin to catch yourself in the grips of an emotional eating episode and become familiar enough with it to start observing yourself with some perspective. Now we want to refine those observations by identifying the *exact* feelings that trigger your emotional eating behavior.

As you learned in part one, emotional eating occurs when you can't face your feelings. Instead, you stuff the feelings down with food. As you already know, you have to hone the skills to accept your feelings, read and interpret what your feelings mean, understand where they lead, and master the art of controlling and regulating the intensity of what you feel without being overwhelmed. When you can do that, you've opened the door to the deeper exploration that we'll go through together.

Four Kinds of Feeling Triggers

There are four different kinds of events that trigger the feelings that make people overeat. Use the lists below to identify the set of feelings that trigger your phantom hunger and uncontrollable urges to eat. You'll be asked first to identify your feelings, and then asked how your feelings relate to your overeating patterns.

EXERCISE
Feeling Trigger #1. Feelings Triggered by Events

Emotionally difficult events trigger uncomfortable feelings. These feelings can be clearly linked to something that happens, whereas other feelings come from relationship friction or are just there.

Below, you'll find a list of potentially volatile events that might activate your feeling phobia. Review the list, checking off any events that have triggered your emotional hunger in the past few months.

List the event and then describe the uncomfortable feelings you had: the ones that made you feel compelled to interrupt the feeling by overeating. We'll call anything that triggers an emotional eating episode a "sore spot."

There's stress or dissatisfaction at work.

I am not focused on something or there's a lull in my day.

I feel challenged or pressured.

The stresses of my life seem totally overwhelming.

There's a lull at work.

I have a free moment at home.

I'm dealing with bills or financial problems.

I have to work too long without stopping.

I'm watching television.

I am driving.

I am in a meeting.

I am with my family.

I am in a room full of people.

I am working.

It's cloudy or raining.

I'm under pressure.

I have to take care of someone.

I am alone for too long.

I am forced to be in a room that I find uncomfortable.

I have to do something new.

I'm ready to go to bed.

Demands are made by my children or family.

I have a sick parent.

I have an unsympathetic spouse.

I have financial burdens (mortgages or taxes).

Example: "When I'm dealing with my sick parent, it makes me feel exhausted. After getting back from the hospital, I can't stop myself from bingeing."

EXERCISE
Feeling Trigger #2: Feelings Triggered by a Person

Uncomfortable feelings come most frequently from friction in relationships. Use the list below to identify what has happened to you recently to trigger an overeating episode by completing the statement below. With whom did you have this friction, and what did you feel? Go through the list and check off the three most relevant sore spots.

"I get set off and want to overeat when someone _____."

criticizes me	betrays me
misunderstands me	smothers me
judges me	deprives me of material things
manipulates me	takes their anger out on me
accuses me	neglects me
ignores me	competes with me
embarrasses me	ridicules me
discourages me	treats me like a child
compares me to others	threatens me
withdraws love from me	rebels against me
invades my privacy	lies to me
doesn't trust me	pressures me
underestimates me	takes me for granted
opposes me	clings to me
expects me to be perfect	scolds me
wants me to feel guilty	excludes me

overprotects me	talks down to me
doesn't respect me	intimidates me
blames me	is unfaithful to me
overindulges me	overpowers me
scapegoats me	insults me
disappoints me	insists on their way

Take the three sore spots you chose and write down how each makes you feel initially and what it provokes in you that makes you want to eat.

Example: "When I feel rejected by my boyfriend, it makes me feel angry as well as jealous of my sister, who is happily married. That combination of jealousy and anger makes me eat."

EXERCISE

Feeling Trigger #3: Feelings Triggered by Unprovoked Feelings

Another set of feelings might arise in the aftermath of events and friction in relationships, rather than at the time of the occurrence. You might become aware of these feelings during an interlude from your daily activities. These feelings are the result of your brain trying to understand what is happening in your life and making assessments of where you are and what is real or not real.

Look at the list below. This is a list of feelings rather than events or people that trigger feelings. You might need to ponder some to determine just what set off these feelings—that's the point of this exercise.

Review this list to pinpoint some of the feelings that are likely to trigger your strong desire to eat something quickly. Try to tie the emotion to the time and circumstance during which this feeling occurs.

Example: "Sometimes late at night when no one is around, I feel lonely and have to eat something."

depressed	jealous	bored
frustrated	lonely	ashamed

anxious   humiliated   needy

angry   uncomfortable   empty

overwhelmed   guilty   scared

afraid   confused

EXERCISE

Feeling Trigger #4: Feelings Triggered by Self-Doubts

As you know from part one, each of us has particular vulnerabilities that trigger our worst thoughts about ourselves. This fourth set of feelings is a special category, and we'll be working with it throughout the entire program of *Shrink Yourself*. You'll recognize it as the first layer of powerlessness: the self-doubt layer. Here all you need to do is identify which of the self-doubt labels listed below you tend to give yourself when you are your own worst, most unforgiving, and harshest critic. This is everyone's weak spot, and is one of the main factors that keeps the feeling phobia alive.

Use this list to identify the three most relevant self-doubt triggers that drive your urge to eat.

"I find I need to eat when I believe I'm _____."

powerless   childish

unlovable   totally lacking warmth or
                                            tenderness
hopeless
                                        lacking courage or strength
self-destructive
                                        lacking talent or abiltiy
untrustworthy
                                        lacking what it takes to deal
inferior   with people

mean and cruel   unable to live up to reason-
                                            able expectations
unworthy
                                        unable to make or keep a
disobedient   commitment

defective or damaged in   dependent
    some way

not a whole person

stupid	helpless
self-centered	too meek
not feminine enough	bad
not masculine enough	alone
not self-sufficient	boring
	weak
	other _____ (specify)

Example: "I find I need to eat when I believe I'm unlovable. In those moments I go to the kitchen and eat whatever I can find."

Now you've identified feelings that trigger your emotional eating in each of these four categories. These are the four different ways that an emotional eating episode begins. Don't worry about the overlaps that inevitably happen in real life. We chose these four categories so it'll be easier to analyze why you have to run away from these feelings.

Identify Your Catastrophe Predictions

As we pointed out in part one, it's the catastrophe predictions that we make when we feel something (angry, hurt, rejected) that make the feelings seem impossible to bear, which of course creates the feeling phobia. The catastrophe predictions the feelings evoke leave us overwhelmed. We say things to ourselves like: "When I am criticized I feel like I will 'explode,' 'evaporate,' 'disintegrate,' or not be able to handle the emotion in some other way." "When I feel betrayed I feel like I'll never be able to trust anyone again."

These catastrophe predictions are not necessarily accurate, but you need to prove that to yourself by using the following lists to connect the feelings you have identified to the catastrophe predictions you're making. It's your turn to see how you're turning your feelings into catastrophe predictions. We'll do this for all four types of feelings discussed above.

EXERCISE

Catastrophe Prediction #1: Catastrophe Predictions for Feelings Triggered by Events

The reason people are afraid to stick with these feelings has mostly to do with being overwhelmed or flooded. No matter which events or feelings you wrote down, see if one of the following fears is lurking in the back of your mind.

It's just too much for me to handle; I'll fall apart.

This is just the beginning of a deluge of problems that will swamp me.

This is a sign that my life is going to fall apart.

I am being tested and I am going to fail.

If this keeps up, I will just give up and curl up into a ball.

I give up; it's just too much stress.

I have to run away as fast as I can.

Take the example that you wrote for this category and tack on one of the lines above.

Example: "When I'm dealing with my sick parent, it makes me feel exhausted. On the drive home from the hospital I start to think that *it's just too much for me to handle and that I'll fall apart.* When I get home, I can't stop myself from bingeing."

EXERCISE

Catastrophe Prediction #2: Catastrophe Predictions for Feelings Triggered by Relationships

This is the same exercise as above. We'll be repeating it for each of the types of feelings and the catastrophe predictions that you create for each. The catastrophe predictions that accompany the feelings triggered by relationship friction have to do with the outcome of that relationship. Here is a list of predictions. Ask yourself which one of these catastrophe predictions you wanted to or needed to banish with food.

"Because of what happened and the way I felt, I was afraid that unless I interrupted or got rid of my feelings _____."

I would lash out in anger.

I would burst out in tears.

I would say or do something I would regret.

I would melt into a puddle.

I would feel guilty forever.

I would never trust again.

I would lose the relationship.

I would quit or be fired.

I would hurt or damage the person beyond repair.

I would never forgive myself.

Example: "When I feel rejected by my boyfriend, it makes me feel angry as well as jealous of my sister, who is happily married. *I'm afraid I'll lash out in anger at my sister.* That combination of jealousy and anger is what makes me eat. I eat so angry words don't come out."

EXERCISE

Catastrophe Prediction #3: Catastrophe Predictions Triggered by Unprovoked Feelings

Now we want to look at the catastrophe predictions that create a panic mode in those feelings that may not be directly or immediately linked to a specific event or a specific relationship. These are brought about by your unprovoked feelings.

These are the feelings that come up unsolicited and often unwanted, when there are some quiet or alone moments in the car, or at home, or in between tasks at work. They may be hard to grasp at first but grow in intensity and can easily be converted into phantom hunger before you're fully aware of what you're feeling. You have already made a list of these feelings. It's now time for you to explore the catastrophe predictions that frighten you so much you're afraid to feel fully. Some of these unprovoked emotions could be anger or sadness or loneliness, which are all normal feelings, but become problematic when they lead to the catastrophe predictions below and then become too intense to handle. Here is an example. Use your personal experience and choose your own ending.

I'm not as good as I want to be and there's nothing I can do about it.

It'll last forever unless I can figure out a way to get rid of it quickly.

It'll lead to despair or the inability to do anything if I don't stop it quickly.

I'll "explode," "evaporate," "disintegrate," or not be able to handle the emotion in some other way.

My life is ruined. I have screwed up.

I'll never be able to trust anyone again.

I'll never be able to do anything right or ever be successful.

My mind will just stop working and my thinking will never be clear.

There's an endless ocean of tears inside me that will start flowing and never stop.

I'll never be able to make a decision again.

Example: Sometimes late at night when no one is around, I feel lonely. *I believe there is an endless ocean of tears inside me that will start flowing and never stop.* When I have that thought, I have to eat something.

EXERCISE

Catastrophe Prediction #4: Catastrophe Predictions Triggered by Self-Doubts

Let's become acquainted with your catastrophe predictions related to your self-doubt labels. Look at the label, and the next time you're feeling one of these ways about yourself and tempted to eat rather than debate yourself about the issue, see if you are thinking one of these false statements about yourself. If you believe the catastrophe predictions, you have to conclude that you're hopeless and powerless to change. If you question them, you can change all of that.

This is the real me I have been hiding.

If this is what I am, then there is no hope.

This means I am a damaged person and no one will want me.

This makes me unloveable.

This is the reason I have to hide from the world.

There is no fixing this.

A person like this doesn't deserve anything.

Example: I find I need to eat when I believe I'm unloveable. *In that moment I believe that if that's what I am, then there's no hope.* In those moments I go to the kitchen and eat whatever I can find.

Your Catastrophe Predictions

Now you have to convince yourself that these catastrophe predictions won't really happen. These *false* predictions are the tipping point between fear, and comfortable understanding, of your feelings. If you don't examine these thoughts embedded in your feelings (the catastrophe predictions), you'll continue to run away from your feelings because you still believe that something terrible is about to happen. If you examine these catastrophe predictions, you'll learn that nothing terrible is going to happen, which means you'll be able to handle adverse events much better in the future without having to interrupt your feelings with food.

Here's what happens: Something occurs. You start to feel intensely about it, and then go into a panic mode, thinking something terrible is going to happen (like you're going to fall apart or run away). These are images in your mind. These are predictions that make you so afraid that you want to stuff something in your mouth immediately because the act of doing so interrupts the horrible feeling. Every time you interrupt the feeling because you're afraid of the catastrophe prediction that accompanies it, you reinforce your fear. This is the vicious cycle that prevents you from learning a better way of dealing with your intense feelings.

You have to demonstrate to yourself that you can quiet your own mind, that you can rise above the moment to get a perspective on yourself and see that you have other options besides eating. You have within yourself a mature response to handling the stressors in life with wisdom. If you can prove to yourself that intense feelings aren't going to destroy you, then you won't panic every time you begin to feel something.

EXERCISE

Reinterpreting Your Catastrophe Predictions: A Reality Check

If you master the catastrophe predictions in all four types of feelings, you'll get rid of your feeling phobia. Then you'll be free to feel your feelings, sort them out, and analyze them. That opens the door to your interior life, which will lead to a better understanding of yourself and of the world you live in. Your feelings can resume their part of your own natural flow of information, and you'll make better and wiser decisions in how you conduct your life, and better responses to specific people and specific situations. But even more immediately, it will allow you to analyze and reverse the powerlessness that drives you to food.

It's food that keeps these catastrophe predictions reinforced and intact because you use food to banish your fears. You need to observe and learn for yourself that these false predictions, if you stay with and understand them, are actually useless and vacant ideas that you can easily discard.

Let's take the examples we've worked with so far in this chapter, and see how being aware of the catastrophe prediction will make it easier to avoid food. Note that the catastrophe predictions are in italic.

Powerless Choice #1

When I'm dealing with my sick parent it makes me feel exhausted. On the drive home from the hospital I start to think that *it's just too much for me to handle and that I'll fall apart*. When I get home, I can't stop myself from bingeing.

Powerful Reinterpretation   I stop and analyze my catastrophe prediction. I realize that it *is* a lot for me to handle right now, but it's not going to be this way forever. When I'm able to do that, the urge to eat decreases.

Powerless Choice #2

When I feel rejected by my boyfriend, it makes me feel angry as well as jealous of my sister, who is happily married. *I'm afraid I'll lash out in anger at my sister*. That combination of jealousy and anger is what makes me eat. I eat so angry words don't come out of my mouth.

Powerful Reinterpretation   When I stop and look at my catastrophe prediction, I realize that my relationship with my boyfriend has nothing to do with my sister. Once I realize that I'm still angry but don't have to be afraid of lashing out at my sister because of my own problems, I don't need food. I can think of other things to do with my angry feelings.

Powerless Choice #3

Sometimes late at night when no one is around, I feel lonely. *I believe there is an endless ocean of tears inside me that will start flowing and never stop*. When I have that thought I have to eat something.

Powerful Reinterpretation   I stop and look at my catastrophe prediction and realize that anytime I've cried in the past, I usually feel better once the tears stop. Maybe it wouldn't be so bad to have a good cry and realize that being home alone is in fact hard.

Powerless Choice #4

I find I need to eat when I believe I'm unloveable. *In that moment I believe that if that's what I am, then there's no hope.* In those moments I go to the kitchen and eat whatever I can find.

Powerful Reinterpretation   If I stop and look at my catastrophe prediction, I can see that I'm *feeling* unloveable, but I'm not really unloveable. It's not who I've always been and it's not who I'm going to always be. Maybe there's something else I can do right now to remind myself that I'm not really unloveable.

By the examples above perhaps you can see how looking at your catastrophe predictions in a fair and analytical way can weaken your urgent need to overeat.

12

SESSION 3
Waking Up from the Food Trance

Food provides you a way to feel better, at least temporarily. People report that they eat when they're sad, angry, bored, or lonely; it doesn't really matter what the feeling is, because having intense feelings is uncomfortable. When you're in a place where you're afraid of or uncomfortable with your feelings, you stuff food in to banish and control them. There is a spiritual and emotional emptiness that you've been trying to fill with food. Using food this way becomes problematic when it becomes the only source of comfort, the only way to cope with stress or feelings, the only reward you have to give yourself, the only place where you're loved. Food can never replace real love or fulfillment. We all do this occasionally, but if you're reading this book food has probably become your primary mechanism for dealing with feelings and emptiness. You've learned that food is the thing that can help you escape reality and temporarily enter a zone where for a few moments you actually have the illusion of well-being. That's the essence of the food trance I described in chapter 2: "While I'm eating nothing can harm me, I feel safe, like I'm in a bubble." What food actually provides is this: when you eat to banish an uncomfortable feeling, you're interrupting the feeling.

And when you enter the food trance, you're replacing the feeling with the temporary bliss that the food trance provides. The food trance is the other side of the feeling phobia coin. Interrupting your feelings with food is the feeling phobia; the bliss that food provides to replace the pain of bad feelings is the food trance.

Starting Point: How to Work with Your Sore Spots

In the last chapter, you looked at events, people, feelings, and self-doubts that triggered you to overeat. We're calling these your sore spots. I'd like you to take two or three of them and work with them in the exercises below. Write them down in your notebook.

EXERCISE

The Escape That the Food Trance Provides

Example: "When I'm at work (event sore spot), I feel bored (feeling). I believe I'll never get a job that satisfies me (catastrophe prediction). I want to eat something quickly (feeling phobia), so I go to the vending machine and get a bag of chips. While I'm eating, a rational calmness comes over me (food trance)."

"While I'm eating to escape the intensity of my negative feelings, I feel _____."

a rational calmness

like I'm in a drug fog

like I'm in a place to feel good

like I have time with a friend who is always there for me

like I have a reminder of a time with my mother

like I'm in a safe bubble where no harm can touch me

like I'm in a place where there are no demands or expectations

like I'm in a place where I'm loved the way my parents never loved me like I'm in a place where I'm trying to be perfect

like I have a complete change of focus away from the real world

like I'm in a place where no one can reach me

EXERCISE

Words That Describe the Rewards
of Being in the Food Trance

"When I'm in the food trance, I feel _____."

rewarded	content	capable
in control	relaxed	complete
confident	calm	comfortable
safe	powerful	nurtured
secure	independent	happy
numb	pleasured	free
satisfied	completely focused on the tastes	

When you make your observations, try to capture the unique experience of being in a food trance as we described it in chapter 2. The list above is just words on paper. The real phenomenon is a state of mind, a bubble of well-being, a time-out—a disconnect from reality. Try to capture that and put it into your own words if you can. Include selections from the list above to get you started. Being able to switch to a new state of mind is a very powerful motive to continue your emotional eating pattern, so get to know your seductress as well as you can.

EXERCISE

Understanding the Vicious Cycle

There are short- and long-term ways that the food trance hurts you. The short-term ways are perhaps more obvious: overeating in order to go into the food trance makes you gain weight and feel guilty, and means you can never control your weight.

I've asked you to observe yourself in several ways so far: observe the feelings that trigger your compulsion to overeat, the catastrophe predictions that keep your feeling phobia intact, and the reward you give yourself temporarily in the form of a food trance. We can now add the way you punish yourself after a binge.

Here's what that looks like when it is all put together in one picture: "When I'm feeling betrayed (trigger), I feel like I'll never have anyone who loves me in my life (catastrophe prediction). I sit down with a pint of ice cream (feeling phobia) and for the few moments that it takes to eat it, I am in a bubble (food trance). I don't feel unworthiness. I just concentrate on the creamy sweetness of the food. But when it's done, I no longer just feel betrayed, but now I hate myself for being so weak (cost of the food trance). How could anyone be true to someone as weak as me (eating actually confirms original trigger)?"

Now put your own statement together so you can understand how the combination of your feelings and catastrophe predictions incite you to eat because you want to replace those uncomfortable feelings with the good feelings of the food trance. Use the example above to add what happens to you after the food trance. Do you feel disgust, guilt, self-hatred, or disappointment? This should illustrate how destructive the vicious cycle of overeating is to your emotional well-being. The short-term cost of the food trance is that you feel guilty, but the long-term cost is that it stops you from being able to grow as a person.

See What You're Trying to Escape

Remember that the feeling phobia and the food trance are two parts of the same strategy: to run away from, rather than learn from, what's going on inside you. Here are some of the things you are trying to escape from:

1. *Events and Stressors: Real-Life Issues*
   The food trance is just another way to delay dealing with the frictions of life that are creating all the feelings you're trying to run away from.

2. *Real-Life Relationship Tension*
   The food trance is just another way to delay dealing with the real issues in your relationships that are creating all the feelings you're trying to run away from.

3. *Intensity of Feelings*
   Being in the food trance gives you a replacement feeling for the panic feeling of your catastrophic predictions. The food trance is a way to dial down the intensity of a feeling.

4. *Self-Doubts*
   The food trance is a way to deal with self-doubts because the idea of facing your self-doubts is so overwhelming and you don't yet know how to deal with them.

Alternatives to Escaping into the Food Trance

Although the food trance exerts a powerful pull that's hard to resist when emotions assail you, you're hardly helpless. You don't have to keep repeating the overeating pattern that has you entrapped. From now on, your work will be to figure out alternatives to the emotional eating pattern. You'll see that:

1. You can address the offending situation directly. If a problem arises at work, for instance, you can talk to your boss instead of eating, you can quit, you can ask for a transfer, you can resolve to try harder—you have options other than hitting the vending machine. Or if your spouse disappoints you, you can talk it over, you can get counseling, you can move out, you can recognize your own contribution to the difficulty. One thing's for sure: overeating won't rescue you from any problem on this earth.

2. You can examine what you need to do in the real world to get your needs met in a substantial way. You've been using food to achieve the happy feeling states you identified a few pages back—eating to make yourself feel contented, safe, or whatever.

You can achieve those same emotional states without food if you do the work to figure out how.

3. You can battle with your inner critic to prevent self-lacerating verdicts about yourself from holding sway over your life.

4. You can engage in concrete activities other than eating to relieve emotional intensity—activities far more healthful than overindulgence.

The first three options above require more work. We'll deal with those in later sessions. Right now we're going to start with the fourth option by identifying strategies that will help you continue your journey without resorting to binges. These represent the choices that everyone else uses to deal with the stressors of life if food has not become their source of comfort. The choices below will give you a time-out so that the intensity of the feeling can lessen a bit and you can think more clearly.

Begin by keeping in mind the three sore spots you selected, then identify a series of specific techniques you can use to relieve emotional pressure before you find your face in a bag of chips.

Choose Your Interventions

Please choose three techniques from each category so you'll have an arsenal of strategies at your command to use whenever intense and frightening emotions wash over you. Then you can choose to intervene before succumbing to your cravings, and you'll never again be able to say to yourself, "What else could I do?" These are the choices that you'll use when you feel sore spots that trigger you to eat.

EXERCISE

How to Dial Down the Intensity of Your Feelings

The goal is to create a mental space so that you have the time to sort out, think, make reinterpretations, and get a new perspective. Then you can disprove your catastrophe predictions, and that will open the door to your interior life. The following things are not difficult to do. In fact, many people who don't struggle with their weight do these things effortlessly. It's just that, for you, you've come to believe that food is the most effective way to dial down the intensity of your feelings.

Relaxation

Select three relaxation strategies from the list.

"To deal with intense feelings without food, I can relax. More specifically, I can _____."

practice deep breathing

practice meditation

take a long hot bath

get a massage

use tension-releasing techniques

use biofeedback techniques

use aromatherapy

take a sauna or a steambath

practice visualization techniques

listen to relaxation tapes

listen to soothing music

spend time in nature

spend time reading

spend time with pets

just hang out and do nothing

go for a walk

watch television or a movie

take a nap

other _____ (specify)

Have More Fun

Select three fun strategies from the list.

"To deal with my intense feelings without food, I can have more fun. More specifically, I can _____."

go to a museum or art gallery

attend a concert, the symphony, or the opera

browse in a bookstore or library

go to the theater

listen to music

attend or watch a sporting event

go to the movies

play a game or cards, or do a puzzle

go shopping

participate in spiritual activities

attend a lecture or seminar

call a good friend

surf the Internet

go on a walk

plan my next vacation

other _____ (specify)

Be More Active

Select three action strategies from the list.

"To deal with my intense feelings without food, I can be more active. More specifically, I can _____."

go running or jogging

take a bike ride

practice yoga

do Pilates

go to the gym

lift weights

work in my garden

go for a walk

play golf

play tennis

participate in other sports

go backpacking, hiking, or camping

practice martial arts

go hunting or fishing

clean the house

other _____ (specify)

Keep Your Perspective

Select three perspective strategies from the list.

"To deal with my intense feelings without food, I can learn to keep my perspective. More specifically, I can _____."

remember a time when I was feeling good

remember what I have to be thankful for

make a plan

remember that I won't always feel this way

remind myself of the people who love or care about me

keep in mind that my life is not as out of control as I think it is

remind myself that my life is not as meaningless as it might feel

let go and remind myself I don't have to control everything

remind myself that what I fear won't necessarily happen

try to help people who are less fortunate than myself

other _____ (specify)

Please record all the strategies you identified in your notebook, and then create a visually appealing list of these strategies to hang on your refrigerator or above your desk. Each time you're faced with an emotional trigger, you will choose one of the corresponding alternatives and then observe what happens to your hunger. It's okay, if you don't avoid eating every time at first.

As you can see, you have a wide array of options other than eating to make yourself feel better. Of course you already knew these strategies, but having them organized in writing may open your eyes to the fact that you can do things other than run to the nearest supermarket when trouble gets you down. The fact that you turn to food before using one of these other strategies indicates that either you don't know how to do something else besides eat, you don't believe that something else will work, or you're afraid to try. Bringing these alternatives to your conscious attention should help you to remember them in the heat of emotional episodes.

Although your impulse still might be to grab a chocolate bar because it's convenient, quick, and immediately gratifying compared to most of the strategies on the list, now you'll know that you can make another choice, and I hope that's what you'll do. After all, the chocolate is gone in a flash and then you're running on empty again.

Remember, you now have two powerful ways to deal with negative feelings other than to binge. First, when catastrophic images arise, you can remember that they are just fears, they are not real, and act accordingly instead of panicking and preparing for the worst. And you can apply strategies from the list you just compiled of mood-controlling actions.

Each time you choose to eat when you're faced with feelings you fear, you'll reinforce your feeling phobia and catastrophe predictions. Each time you use a nonfood way to deal with problems and feelings, you cut the link to using food as a tranquilizer, you get stronger and more powerful, and that's our goal. When you have chosen alternatives to food enough times, your confidence will grow, and food will no longer be the obvious or only choice for how to deal with life.

Deal with Your Feelings without Food

Let's take the examples from the feeling phobia session and see how we can apply the things we learned about the food trance to them:

Powerless Choice #1

When I'm dealing with my sick parent, it makes me feel exhausted. On the drive home from the hospital I start to think that *it's just too much for me to handle and that I'll fall apart.* When I get home, I can't stop myself from bingeing. For a few moments while I'm raiding the refrigerator I forget about the doctor's bills and all the things I need to do. I feel safe and calm, but when the food's gone I not only feel exhausted, I feel disgusted with myself.

Powerful Reinterpretation   When I get home, I draw a bath for myself and call a friend. My friend reminds me that it's not always going to be this way. The bath relaxes me, and I get a good night's sleep. When I wake up I feel better equipped to go back to the hospital.

Powerless Choice #2

When I feel rejected by my boyfriend, it makes me feel angry as well as jealous of my sister, who is happily married. *I'm afraid I'll lash out in anger at my sister.* That combination of jealousy and anger is what makes me eat. I eat so angry words don't come out. I stuff as much food in as possible, and while I'm stuffing I just focus on getting as much food in as fast as I can. While I'm doing this everything else fades away. But when I've eaten everything I can get my hands on and there isn't anything more, I hate myself and think that it's no wonder I don't have a husband like my sister.

Powerful Reinterpretation   When I stop and keep my perspective, I'm able to see that my sister wants me to have a marriage that's as happy as hers. When I remember that she's on my side, I'm not too angry to call her, and she helps me sort out how to talk to my boyfriend.

Powerless Choice #3

Sometimes late at night when no one is around, I feel lonely. *I believe there is an endless ocean of tears inside me that will start flowing and never stop.* When I have that thought I have to eat something. It doesn't matter what time of night it is, I'll go out to 7-Eleven and buy tons of treats and eat them all. Then I feel so disappointed with myself.

Powerful Reinterpretation   When I feel this way I go to Blockbuster and get the sappiest movie I can find. I come home and watch it and let myself cry, and by the time the movie is over, so are the tears, and I actually feel better.

Powerless Choice #4

I find I need to eat when I believe I'm unloveable. *In that moment I believe that if that's what I am, then there's no hope.* In those moments I go to the kitchen and eat whatever I can find. Then, when I stop eating, I feel so angry at myself and I can understand why no one could ever love someone with so little self-control.

Powerful Reinterpretation   I stop and put my sneakers on. I go for a jog, and while I'm running I remember that I only feel unloveable but there are a lot of great things about me, one of them being that even with my extra weight, I can run a solid two miles.

Now that you've exposed and explored your feeling phobia and you've admitted how pleasurable being in the food trance can be, you've reached the goal of these last two sessions and you're ready to look within. With those new eyes, you'll be able to explore the five levels of powerlessness that have been fueling your phantom hunger.

13

SESSION 4
Challenging Your Self-Doubts

In this session:

- You'll see that you have self-doubts. Some are triggered by others, some are unprovoked.

- You'll identify the armor you wear to protect yourself from self-doubts.

- You'll make a reinterpretation that you're in fact powerful in order to deal with your self-doubts.

- You'll learn to dialogue with the six accusations that Harriet makes against you.

- You'll understand that you have two methods of mastering your self-doubts:

  1. You can diminish what's there now by talking back to your nagging critical conscience.

  2. You can stop adding to your load of doubt by catching yourself when you misinterpret a situation to mean there's something wrong with you.

In previous sessions we talked about ways to manage your feeling phobia and food trance without using food. All of the suggestions were meant to provide you with a time-out, another way to step back from what you're feeling in order to dial down the intensity of your emotions. Once the intensity of the feeling is managed, you're more in control and can make better choices. These are short-term solutions, but they're necessary to being able to think clearly. When our minds are more clear, then we can face the real-world problems that need solving and the interior world that needs taming.

We start taming the interior world by listening to, and then talking back to, the voice of the inner critic, Harriet. Remember from part one, *it's the immediate experience of powerlessness that creates the "uncontrollable" urge to eat.* (That's our focus for all the sessions that follow.)

Talk Back to Your Inner Critic

Your self-doubts derive from a history that should be put to rest as you grow up and change. But when you block that from happening by overeating, Harriet pushes PLAY, and the old tape keeps running and is reinforced, harping about the same old shortcomings you suffered from at age five or ten or fifteen, except that the voice is no longer a critical parent or teacher, the voice is your own and lives inside you. I'm not saying that you've become perfect, by any means, but I'm willing to bet that most of the deep-seated negative attitudes you have about yourself are exaggerated. We know that these self-doubts are the first interior destination of powerlessness that you fear, and as long as you're afraid to face them, you'll continue to be addicted to escaping into your feeling phobia and food trance. Therefore, it's critically important that you look at, rather than away from, your self-doubts.

You need to make a good assessment of yourself, discover the truth, and figure out what to do, other than eat pizza, when the self-doubt music plays. In this session we'll start this critical work (work that all successful, fulfilled human beings must do) and we'll confront your inner critic.

- Listen to and analyze what your critical self is saying. You can talk back only if you listen first.

- Learn new ways to effectively talk back to the six accusations Harriet makes.

    1. If you're not perfect, you're deeply flawed.

    2. You're trying to cover up and deny your real faults.

    3. You're a phony.

    4. You're a pretend adult and don't deserve the full rights of adulthood.

    5. You know the good stuff about you isn't real.

    6. Everybody knows what you're hiding.

- Learn how to stop reinforcing the powerlessness conclusion that something is wrong with you.

When you tell someone that their hair looks great, they usually don't say "Thank you," they usually say "Really? But it's dirty" or "No, it doesn't." People desperately want to be validated, seen, known, appreciated, and acknowledged, yet they're so eager to convince you of what's wrong with them. Harriet has whole lists of criticisms that she waits to deploy in your direction the minute life doesn't go your way. So I'd like to give you the opportunity to tell us what's really wrong with you. You might be saying, "Wait, this book is supposed to help me with my self-esteem, not convince me of all the horrible things I already believe about myself." Well, I once heard a comedienne say, "You know how when you tell someone you don't like them, you kind of start to like them a little bit." If you can be up front and almost have a sense of humor about what you don't like about yourself, you'll come out of hiding and those self-doubts will get less frightening.

EXERCISE

What's Wrong with You?

Here is the same list of self-doubts you looked at in Session 2. These are the things that Harriet calls you. Select the ones you identify with.

"I think I'm _____."

defenseless	not self-sufficient
unloveable	childish
hopeless	coldhearted
untrustworthy	cowardly
inferior	talentless
mean	incapable
cruel	unreliable
unworthy	too dependent
disobedient	helpless
defective	too meek
damaged	bad
incomplete	totally alone
stupid	boring
self-centered	weak
unfeminine	pathetic
unmasculine	

Now, let's make them specific. That's where you'll really see how cruel you let Harriet be to you. Write a narrative around your self-doubt label. Here's a couple of examples.

James, thirty-nine, is a musician. He's had dreams of being a rock star for twenty years. In addition to his regular gigs, which don't make him much money, he has started to play music for children in a preschool. He still depends on his mother to give him $1,000 a month to meet his expenses. Harriet tells him, "You're pathetic." Whenever he goes to family functions, he doesn't connect with his brothers or brothers-in-law, who are all younger but able to support themselves, so he barely participates in any conversations. Instead, he plays with the kids in the yard and ends up hiding out at the dessert table. Stuffing himself with sweets makes him feel even more pathetic.

Dora, a fifty-six-year-old woman whose children are grown and live scattered throughout the country, has no job and no real interests of her own. Harriet convinces her that she's all alone and boring. She wouldn't dare put expectations on her children, but she doesn't know how to go out and meet new people on her own. Most days she sits at home with her disabled husband, retreats into books, and has an all-day grazing session. Harriet's right: she's virtually all alone and she is boring.

Defend Yourself against Harriet's Accusations

The question "What's wrong with you?" deals with the first two accusations Harriet makes against you.

Accusation #1: If you're not perfect, you're deeply flawed.

Accusation #2: You're trying to cover up and deny your real faults.

If you've identified a self-doubt you want to work on today and have marshaled all the evidence you can to prove to the invisible jury that you're guilty as charged, then you're ready to take over the defense's side. Here you'll practice ways to talk back to Harriet, the prosecutor.

Let's see what James and Dora could've said back to Harriet when she called them names.

Defense to Accusation #1: If you're not perfect, you're deeply flawed

When Harriet tells you you're not perfect and therefore you're deeply flawed, you don't have to accept it, you can talk back to her. You could say one of the following things:

- It's okay to have limitations.
- I can't expect to know everything.

- I can't control every situation.
- I can't expect to perfectly control myself.
- Not everyone can love me the way I want to be loved.
- I can't expect to perform perfectly.
- No one is perfect.
- Just because I can't do something right doesn't mean I can't do anything right.
- Just because I made mistakes in the past doesn't mean I won't do things better in the future. It's okay to have limitations.

We all have flaws. No matter how much it might seem so from the outside, no one is perfect.

James, for example, could have a conversation with Harriet. Let's see what that might look like.

Harriet: You're pathetic taking money from your mother at thirty-nine. When are you going to grow up?

James: You're right. I wish I didn't need to take money from her. But I'm a late bloomer and just because I can't do something right (support myself fully) doesn't mean I can't do anything right. I'm creating new work opportunities for myself every day.

Harriet: Who are you kidding? When are you going to grow up?

James: This year, I'm taking half the money I took from her last year. Maybe, at this rate, by next year I'll barely need any money from her at all.

Harriet: You'll still have to be ashamed of all the years you did take money from her.

James: You know what, Harriet, I'm just going to accept that my path looks different than my brothers' and my brothers-in-law's. I'm not going to feel bad about it anymore. I'm going to keep working hard and let my mother know how much I appreciate the support she's been giving me. I really believe I won't need it for much longer.

James finds that when he simply accepts his situation and is grateful to his mother, he no longer needs to be sheepish at family functions. He can actually participate with the adults and engage in conversation. He discovers that when he's doing that, he forgets all about the dessert table.

Take your self-doubt from the list on page 199. If it falls into a category where Harriet is convincing you that because you're not perfect, you're deeply flawed, then have a dialogue with her like James did above.

Defense to Accusation #2: You're trying to cover up and deny your real faults

> It is rewarding to find someone you like, but it is essential to like yourself. It is quickening to recognize that someone is a good and decent human being, but it is indispensable to view yourself as acceptable. It is a delight to discover people who are worthy of respect and admiration and love, but it is vital to believe yourself deserving of these things.—*Jo Coudert*

Remember the catastrophe predictions that perpetuated the feeling phobia? Those messages made you fear your own emotions as if they were huge, destructive forces that could destroy you and other people, instead of recognizing them as important communications that deserved to be heeded. You might have a similar fear of your own faults. You might be scared to death about admitting any faults, worrying that they indicate some awful, huge, shameful truth about you. This attitude is just plain wrong, harsh, and even silly, and it paralyzes you needlessly.

Every human on earth has faults. The task of growing up means that you need to accept this and understand that you are, in fact, an imperfect human being figuring it out as you go along—just like everyone else. That's the life cycle perspective versus the childhood perspective. The life cycle perspective assumes that you're an adult navigating through a complex and sometimes dangerous world, a person who has to be alert and adaptive, and who must continue to learn in order to flourish. The childhood perspective clings to the vestiges of an illusion that you can measure your behavior by a simple formula, a formula learned in childhood and endowed with the authority of parents who know best. This formula can't be questioned because dropping it means losing the security provided by believing in the illusion of one right authority who has the virtue of being familiar and known, no matter how harsh that authority is.

To recover from childhood, you need to stop automatically believing Harriet, accepting when Harriet accuses you that the accusation is either all right or all wrong. You need to develop discrimination and free your ability to think creatively for yourself, to think about truth and degrees, rather than pronouncements and absolutes. These abilities come as the result of a lot of wrestling with Harriet. You need to have ongoing, multilevel dialogues with her in order to see your problems in perspective and to empower yourself to do something other than accepting a first-round verdict without sifting through the evidence and granting yourself proper appeals. If every therapist accepted all the horrible things that their patients were saying about themselves as truth, they would never make any progress. You must be your own therapist and figure out what part of the story Harriet is leaving out. What could Dora have told Harriet when Harriet accused her of being all alone and boring?

Harriet: Dora, you're all alone and boring. Your kids have all moved away. They don't want to be around you.

Dora: Just because they don't live around me doesn't mean they don't love me. I did a good job raising them, and now they're confident enough to be on their own.

Harriet: But you're boring. You don't do anything all day except read mystery novels and play Sudoku.

Dora: You're right. I have been sitting around just passing time. It doesn't mean I'm boring, though. I've just forgotten who I am now that I'm not so busy taking care of the kids. I was actually a really great mother, I did a lot of creative things with the kids, and I bet I could apply those things to my own life now. By the way, Harriet, thanks for pointing out that I haven't been using my talents as well as I could be. By the way, can you play Sudoku? It's really quite challenging.

Once Dora has admitted that the fault Harriet pointed out actually has some truth to it, Harriet is left speechless. When you have your dialogue with Harriet, you are representing the real world of today while she is representing the world of yesterday. Just as I don't allow myself to be convinced by all of my patients' self-doubts, you can't be convinced by Harriet's.

EXERCISE ARMOR

Preparation for Defense to Accusation #3

Most people are other people. Their thoughts are someone else's opinions, their lives a mimicry, their passions a quotation.
—*Oscar Wilde,* De Profundis, *1905*

As we alluded before, your self-doubts may make you so uncomfortable that you need to retreat into a sort of "armor" to avoid feeling bad about yourself. By retreating into some sort of role, you distance yourself from the pain of feeling like a failure. Review the list of typical "armor roles" below. Which of these roles do you adopt when your self-doubt is activated? Write the ones that most closely align with your own defense system in your notebook and reflect on how adopting these roles has affected your growth and happiness in your relationships and throughout your life.

dreamer	bully
busy person	expert
loner	leader
workaholic	procrastinator
perfectionist	victim
people-pleaser	seducer/seductress

clown	freewheeler
self-indulger	complainer
martyr	someone who needs nobody
indifferent person	competitor
noncompetitor	party animal
logician	apologizer
controller	dropout
liar	mother

Realize that you've adopted these roles to compensate for or to master a lack of confidence. Pick out one or two of your armor roles. You may use many, but for now pick the ones that you know cause you problems with others or that limit you in some definite way. Now try to identify what self-doubt you're covering up by the use of these exaggerated roles (the armor roles are usually natural strengths being overused to create a protective shell around yourself). Wearing the armor can become so habitual that you mistake the alias for your true self. However you've handled Harriet, your inner critic up until now, it's likely that you've addressed your lack of confidence indirectly, which isn't the best way to rid yourself of it. And so it's useful to identify the type of armor you wear so that you can begin stepping out of it to address your self-doubt head-on. Maybe by now you can see that you haven't been presenting a false front, but overusing a true strength.

Amy has always enjoyed being alone. Her parents said she used to spend hours in her room caught up in an imaginative world of play. While Amy's capacity to spend time alone in a productive way is something that she likes about herself, lately she's been using it as a cover-up. She is an artist who paints for many hours in her studio. While she's painting she tends to snack on Gummi Bears and soda. She's gained thirty pounds in the past year. She tells everyone she's just so busy preparing for her gallery opening that she can't socialize anymore. But in reality, she doesn't want anyone to see how much weight she's gained. She's hiding behind her loner armor.

Defense to Accusation #3: You're a phony

Harriet will try to accuse you of being a phony because you've been wearing your armor. She doesn't have compassion for the fact that the only reason you've been wearing it is because you felt inadequate in some way. What will you tell her when she says you're a phony? Let's see what Amy told her:

> *Harriet:* Amy, you're a phony. You're not really an artist who needs to be alone. You're hiding out because you're afraid to take risks to meet people, and you know they're going to think you're fat now that you've gained weight.

> *Amy:* No, Harriet, I actually do like being alone, but you're right that I've been alone more than I want to be lately.

> *Harriet:* You don't even know who you are underneath that armor.

> *Amy:* I do know who I am. I'm an artist, and I like my work, and I'm trying my best. I'm just afraid no one will love the me that's underneath this armor.

> *Harriet:* Well, you're too chicken to even put yourself out there to see if they might.

> *Amy:* You're right. Up until now I have been, but I've taken lots of risks with my art and I've been well received. Maybe I can take some risks with people, too.

When you admit that you've just been wearing your armor because you're scared, Harriet probably won't provide you with the compassion you want or need. But you can provide it for yourself by understanding that underneath that heavy armor is a pretty remarkable person.

Defense to Accusation #4: You're a pretend adult, and don't deserve the full rights of adulthood

Harriet tries to convince you that you're still a child because only when you believe that you're a child does she have any power over you. You'll have to watch for self-defeating behavior patterns that you fall into at the moment when the self-doubt first arises, behaviors that actually keep you acting like a child. Do any of the patterns below describe your behavior when you experience self-doubt?

You're responding to Harriet whenever you find yourself behaving in any of the following ways.

- becoming very intimidated and caving in or holding your opinion back
- acting as if other people must be right and you must be wrong
- feeling afraid to express your feelings
- feeling guilty, as if you've done something wrong
- forgetting your basic rights and not feeling entitled to anything
- being afraid to show your potential, true competency, or talent

These are all the self-defeating behaviors that are based on the premise that you're not a fully enfranchised adult person with a voice who deserves whatever luck or hard work or opportunity can offer. Every time you act this way you reenforce Harriet's power because you're agreeing with her that you're an undeserving person. Your actions in the real world are mistakenly based on your acceptance of Harriet's view of the world—a misinterpretation.

Your dialogue with Harriet on this issue is not with words or self-talk. It's with action. You have to do the opposite of the behaviors on the list above. For example, if you're afraid to express your feelings, you need to find a way to express them. You're an adult now, and this is your right. Every time you take an action that contradicts something on the list above, you'll be weakening Harriet and strengthening yourself.

Defense to Accusation #5: You know the good stuff about you isn't real

> Stop all this self-flagellation and let's get on with it. We've got a world to change.—*Neale Donald Walsch,* CWG Bulletin

Now you need to prepare for Harriet's most devious assault of all. She doesn't bother to accuse you of anything, she just makes you feel undeserving, as if there is some good reason you shouldn't have everything you can have in life. Self-doubt can make you forget that you have any redeeming qualities at all. You might have just received an Oscar or an Emmy, but if self-doubt attacks, you'll find a way to feel lousy anyway. You could, for instance, convince yourself that if the panel of judges knew the truth about you, they would have chosen someone else, or you could tell yourself that the award applies to your former self, not to the you of today. As you already know, self-doubt can make you feel that you have nothing at all to offer to anyone or to the world around you.

One way to interrupt a self-doubt hurricane is to simply keep a positive frame of mind and remember times when you were proud of yourself or just happy to be you. It's a simple and obvious technique, but it truly can help to recall your good qualities if you keep them before you. But Harriet has a counterattack planned, so you'll have to be on guard. She knows how to disconnect her world and your world so that everything good about you doesn't count in her world. You may be fantastic in every way, but she won't let you be happy. My patient Lauren said, "When things happen at my school where I'm a teacher or with my friends, I immediately think the worst no matter what is actually going on. My co-teacher might say something nice, my students might hug me and tell me how great they think I am, I am always shown how well-liked I am, and yet I am so far into my own thoughts and paranoia that I make myself feel completely worthless. No amount of validation on anybody's part makes a dent in how I feel about myself."

Let's see what Lauren could've told Harriet every time Harriet tried to discount her accomplishments.

Harriet: You know the good stuff about you isn't real. You aren't really a good teacher.

Lauren: You're right, I have doubts about my teaching, but I'm convinced by the responses that I'm getting, the feedback from my co-teacher, and the hugs from my students that my doubts aren't necessarily true.

Harriet: They're just trying to make you feel good.

Lauren: No, there are too many people telling me the same thing, and I know when someone's just trying to make me feel good, and that's not what's happening. They really mean it, and I've done a lot of good work at my school that I'm proud of. I am a good teacher, but I'm not the best teacher. I'm getting better, so don't try to discount the progress I've made.

Defense to Accusation #6: Everybody knows what you're hiding

Harriet's best trick of all is disguise. Harriet can migrate. Instead of being a recognizable voice within you, she speaks through your husband or wife, a teacher, someone you thought was your friend, the grocery checkout lady when she seems distant, or anybody that you are afraid to approach and that you expect will be your critic. She actually has you hear what other people are saying as criticism even when it may not be.

Every Hanukah for years Jane and Mark would go to visit Mark's mother. And every year, Mark's mother would ask Jamie, "What did you do with your hair?" Jane would shrug off the question but would feel bad and insecure about her hair for the rest of the evening. Last year, Jane vowed that she would not let this happen again. When she walked into the house, sure enough, Jane's mother-in-law said, "What did you do with your hair?" Jane took a deep breath, paused, and asked "Why do you ask?" Her mother-in-law responded, "Because it looks so lovely." All along Jane had been assuming that her mother-in-law was asking about her hair because there was something wrong with it. Last year was indeed different. Jane didn't feel bad about herself all night, and the family had a nice dinner. This year Jane is actually looking forward to seeing her mother-in-law for the holiday.

When you see Harriet in others, you take one or two approaches. You give them all of Harriet's power and either avoid them or appease them—anything so you won't be attacked. The other approach is to fight back: They are dead wrong. You're absolutely right. It's a win/lose battle, and you are not going to lose. But of course you lose automatically when you confuse the real issues and frictions in daily life that have to be resolved with this fight to the death to defend your honor and battle with the person who only represents Harriet at the moment. It's a surefire way to lose friends, ruin intimacy, and become an isolated, misunderstood person, all of which make Harriet's other assaults on you stronger.

Let's see how Jane was able to dialogue with Harriet and have a breakthrough with her mother-in-law.

Harriet: Everyone knows what you're hiding, especially your mother-in-law.

Jane: I see you out there, Harriet, and I'm not going to talk to you when you're in that disguise.

Harriet: Your mother-in-law thinks you're awful and you're not good enough for her son.

Jane: She's never said that.

Harriet: But she thinks it. You know it, I know it, Mark knows it, everyone knows it.

Jane: I'm not listening to you anymore. I'm just going to ask her myself.

As you know, Jane did ask her mother-in-law why she always asked about her hair, and she discovered that it was actually because she liked it, not because she was judging her. Being able to identify how Harriet is operating in the people around you frees you up to have real relationships with those people. Just like a good therapist, you will do some detective work to see what role Harriet is playing in your challenging relationships.

Stop Reinforcing Your Powerlessness

With regard to your self-doubts, making a powerless choice looks like this:

Something happens. There's a situation (below are a few exam-ples, but I'm sure you can identify what affects you personally in your life) where you feel you're being measured by someone or yourself.

- Someone makes a comment.

- Someone gives you a look.

- You get a poor report at work.

- Someone tells you your child was misbehaving.

When that happens, you begin evaluating your life, your perform-ance, your accomplishments, your love life. You arrive at the misin-terpretation that there's something wrong with you. Your self-doubts make you feel powerless, and you eat, seeking refuge in the food trance for a few moments. This makes you feel guilty. The whole process confirms your self-doubts. Let's see what this looks like in practice.

Powerless Choice Example

When Alexandra comes home from work, her husband asks, "What are you wearing?" (what happened in the external reality of today). She misinterprets his statement to believe that he's criticizing her outfit. He never likes what she wears; he's not attracted to her. Finally it turns into a catastrophe prediction: He doesn't really love her. She concludes that there's something wrong with her (this hap-pens in her internal reality, where things are weighed against her fears and past experiences). She goes to the kitchen and eats, and when she's done she feels even more full of self-doubt. This experi-ence of eating reinforces both her self-doubts and her experience of powerlessness.

Powerful Reinterpretation   When something happens, you have two choices: you can dialogue with Harriet or you can evaluate the situ-ation based on what is happening today. You can see if the negative evaluation that you assume someone has made against you is accurate

downright wrong

exaggerated

politically motivated

an example of how a person is dumping on you

perhaps partly true, but doesn't mean that's the only truth about
you

Powerful Reinterpretation Example   When Alexandra comes home
from work, her husband asks, "What are you wearing?" She thinks
about what's really going on. He asked her a question, nothing
more. She evaluates what could be going on. Maybe he's never seen
the outfit; maybe he's wondering why she's so dressed up since it's
casual Friday. There's no way for her to know what he meant and so
she doesn't immediately eat, she asks him. If the answer is negative,
she can still weigh his comment against the list above. Perhaps he's
exaggerating; perhaps he doesn't like it when she buys new clothes,
perhaps he just doesn't have the same dress sense as she does. She
doesn't have to conclude that there's something wrong with her
because of the comment her husband made.

14

SESSION 5
Defeat Your Defeatism

In this session:

- You'll learn that the frustration in your life leads you to food as a reward.
- You'll learn that your frustration is based on a false sense of powerlessness. After you learn to recover your agency over your own life, food will have less power over you.
- You'll make whatever changes are necessary to improve your relationships.
- You'll make sure your legitimate needs get met, and that your immature needs are given up.
- You'll take responsibility for your unfulfilled potential.
- You'll take charge of your stress and improve the skills that make that possible.
- You'll learn that you have two methods to recover your power over your own life:
  1. You can proactively deal with your life challenges and make your life work in the areas we've covered.

2. You can avoid defeatism (adding to your false powerless-
    ness) by not letting obstacles and difficulties become rea-
    sons to be a victim of your life, rather than the one in
    charge of it.

We have now looked at the different types of feelings that make
you eat, and what events and which people trigger those feelings.
Now we'll look at the things in your life that are frustrating and disappointing. When you can confront your frustration directly, food
won't seem like the only reward available to you.

Here are four common areas where most people are frustrated:

1. relationships

2. unmet needs

3. unfulfilled potential

4. accumulated stress

There are always things you can do to make your life better
that are not contingent on anyone else. You no longer need to defeat
yourself because you don't do what you can, and if you stop defeating
yourself, you won't have to overeat to feed that emotional hunger.
It's Harriet, your critical conscience, that keeps you from being
the total author and agent of your own life. To get real satisfaction
in life you have to step out of your defeated identity and take real
action.

In the exercises that follow, I am only trying to help you give
yourself some concrete examples of what you can do by making a
decision to do it. I want to remind you that you can choose the powerful pathway in life and be much better off for it. This book alone
cannot "fix" your life, but these exercises can get you going in the
right direction.

EXERCISE

Make Your Relationships Work Better

Here are some specific things you might do to improve a close and
important relationship. Think of a specific person and a recent

incident of friction or disappointment, and ask yourself whether you would have handled it better if you were

trying to open an honest dialogue

expecting less from your partner

accepting that you have different opinions on certain topics

learning not to take certain things so seriously

calling him/her more often

not being so stubborn or hardheaded

not trying to control everything

letting your partner have some space

acknowledging he or she is temporarily under a lot of stress

other _____ (specify)

Observe, Catch Yourself in Mid-Act, and Choose

One way you can improve relationships and diminish emotional hunger is to get real about your relationships—including your expectations of others. Just as you have foibles and they don't add up to the entire you, your partner has foibles that most likely comprise only part of the picture of who he or she is.

If you are frustrated with a relationship, there are things you can do, and they all involve some change in you, your attitude, your behavior, your sensitivity, or your intimacy skills. You need to work on these in order to stop eating. You don't have to solve them all at once, though. Making small changes can actually offer a lot of relief. If you find yourself in a conflict with someone, stop, try to pinpoint what part of the conflict you're responsible for, and choose a different way from the list above to handle it.

EXERCISE

Harriet Checklist

We'll repeat this exercise in each of these four areas in this chapter. It's important for you to see just how pervasive your inner critic is.

You reward yourself with food instead of facing the struggles in your life because of your belief in your defeatism. Your defeatism is based on believing that what Harriet has been saying about you is true—that you're not able to take charge of your life. Pinpoint in what way Harriet is stopping you and then go back to the accusation exercises in Session 4 (chapter 13) and start talking back. Anytime you're convinced that you're ready to try something different or new in your relationships, Harriet has something to say about it.

You say: "In order to improve my relationship with my husband, I can make a request instead of just being angry and disappointed when he doesn't read my mind and do what I want." When you propose that, Harriet says to you one or more of the things from the checklist below in order to defeat you, to stop you from being your own free agent of change:

1. You won't be able to do this perfectly, so you'd better not do it at all. If you do it, you will fail.

2. You have real faults, and everyone will know them if you try to do this. No one will want to be around you or with you.

3. You'll lose your protective armor and be out of control. Anything might happen. (Example: If I stop being a people-pleaser and focus on myself, people won't want to be around me.)

4. You have no right to aspire to anything more than you already have or to speak up for yourself.

5. You'd better not think your accomplishments or the compliments you get prove you're a good person. Don't try to make your life any better.

6. You know who is going to put you down for trying this and what they're going to say about you, so don't even bother.

These six statements that Harriet will make when you try to take action in your life correspond to the six accusations we dialogued with in the last chapter. You'll have to go back to the last chapter and do the accusation exercise for whichever one or ones apply to you with regard to how you deal with your relationships.

Get Your Realistic Needs Met

From the moment we are born, we have needs. We are hungry, we are cold, we're uncomfortable. And as we get older, our list of needs grows more complex and our ability to have them met becomes a real challenge. Part of growing up includes differentiating which needs we can and should be meeting on our own and which can be met only by another person, and how to relate to and share mutually so our needs can be satisfied. Once we've identified this distinction, then we will still have to take responsibility for communicating our needs to those around us and working out a fair and mutual exchange with the others.

EXERCISE
Identify Unmet Needs

Here is a list of legitimate needs that my patients have talked about in our therapy sessions. Think about which of these needs is calling out within you for more satisfaction, or a higher priority, or an absolute demand. Here you will be looking for what you want, whether it is easy to get or not. You will have to know what you want if you are to conquer emotional eating.

Pick out the needs that are at least partially frustrated in your life right now by completing the following sentence:

"I want more _____."

acknowledgment and acceptance

attention and recognition

caring and consideration

challenge and stimulation

closeness and intimacy

financial reward

freedom and personal space

guidance and support

honesty and trust

opportunity for advancement

physical contact and passion

power and status

reliability and stability

respect and appreciation

responsibility and authority

safety and security

sensitivity and communication

sharing and participation

structure and direction

togetherness and belonging

understanding and empathy

other _____ (specify)

You've now completed the first step: acknowledging your needs. Until you admit you have needs, you can't satisfy them. Next you need to separate out realistic from unrealistic needs and identify the specific reasons why you haven't satisfied your realistic needs. That is the analysis you will need in order to make a wise decision about how to get either satisfaction or resolution of your frustrated needs.

Think about one of the needs on your list, then ask yourself Why haven't I satisfied this need yet? You can repeat this for all of the needs if you have time for that. If not, just pick the one that you feel, on a gut level, is the most frustrating to you today, and the most likely to send you looking for a food trance reward.

Example: "I'd like to get my degree, but I have three children and I don't believe it is fair to the family to pursue this now.")

"I have not satisfied this need yet because _____."

it hasn't been a high priority

it's in conflict with another important need (for example, I may want both continuity and change at the same time)

I just haven't figured out how to get this need met

I don't believe it is obtainable in my current situation

I know what I need to do to get this need satisfied, I'm just afraid to try

it may be obtainable, but not worth the effort

I'm afraid to try to satisfy this need because I'll be too stressed trying to get it and too disappointed or depressed if I don't get it

the way I would like this need satisfied is unrealistic (for example, my age, social status, resources, education, or physical health prevent me from being able to do what is necessary to achieve this dream)

to get this need met, I would have to make big changes in my life that I am not now prepared to make

I can get this need met only if someone else will grant it to me or change their behavior or attitude toward me, and I'm not sure I can influence them to do that or I don't know how

I want this need satisfied, but I think I am asking for too much or will never be satisfied no matter how much I get

I want this need satisfied, but it's too unfair to the other people involved to make it happen

Only you know what these answers mean in the fabric of your life, but at least you have a starting point to understand why you have not been able to get this need satisfied. This will start you thinking, and that's what we want: think instead of eat.

Don't Interpret Frustrated Needs to Mean You Are Defeated

As you think about the reasons your frustrated needs have not been satisfied yet, you'll be face to face with your defeatism. Because these needs are not being satisfied, you might be confusing frustration with defeatism, and jumping to the catastrophe prediction that your needs will never get met, ever.

It's more likely that you've made a conscious and deliberate choice not to pursue a specific need satisfaction for one of the reasons above. If that's so, you're not defeated and don't need a reward of extra food to compensate for being a victim. You're not a victim, but in fact, a mature adult. You may have decided the need is not a priority, or that it's a childish wish rather than a mature realizable need, or that it puts other more important needs in jeopardy, or that it's something you'll pursue later rather than now.

As you further explore the need you may finally realize that getting a particular need satisfied is something you want to, should, and will pursue. That's fine, and the same thinking applies: you're not a victim and not defeated, you're just learning more about yourself.

But you may have decided that this is a realizable and important need but that you're in conflict with yourself about getting it satisfied. In that case, you have been defeated by Harriet, and it's Harriet that you have to deal with. If you don't, you'll be left with food as your only possible reward.

Finally, you may decide that what you want is unrealistic, unrealizable, excessive, and maybe even childish or impossible to get. It may even be unwise to get even if you could, like having your partner take care of all the finances that you should really know about yourself. You know you shouldn't lean on other people to do things for you that make you whole, but, rather, you should be developing the mature competency to do those things yourself.

Make Decisions to Become the Agent of Your Own Life

As the agent of your own life, you have to make a highly conscious, thoughtful decision that will put the frustrated need state to rest. There are three possible resting spots, and you won't find full relief from the gnawing aspect of the frustrated need until you arrive at one of them. After minutes, hours, days, weeks, or months, you should have decided on one of the following ways to best handle this need.

1. Try to get my need satisfied more actively, either by my own efforts or by expressing them to someone.

2. Accept a compromised form of this need so I can enjoy what I already have or what is possible.

3. Make a decision that this need can't or shouldn't be fulfilled. Accept that there are other satisfactions in life, so life can go on without feeling deprived and defeated.

Whether you know it or not, you have just outlined a short plan on how to deal with this need. Even if it goes unfulfilled, it won't drive your emotional hunger so strongly because you have decided consciously how to deal with it. Of course, you have to follow through with your plan, but even thinking about needs in this new, open way generally provides most of the relief from emotional hunger.

EXERCISE

Harriet Checklist

Let's pinpoint how Harriet has been playing a role in your frustrated needs. Then go back to the accusation exercises in chapter 13 (Session 4) and start talking back. Anytime you're convinced that you're ready to try to get realistic needs met, Harriet has something to say about it.

You say: "In order to get my need met for more affection, I'm going to initiate sex more often with my partner." When you propose that, Harriet says to you one of the things from the following checklist.

1. You won't be able to do this perfectly, so you'd better not do it at all. If you do it, you will fail.

2. You have real faults, and everyone will know them if you try to do this. No one will want to be around you or with you.

3. You'll lose your protective armor and be out of control. Anything might happen. (Example: If I stop being a people-pleaser and focus on myself, people won't want to be around me.)

4. You have no right to aspire to anything more than you already have or to speak up for yourself.

5. You'd better not think your accomplishments or the compliments you get prove you're a good person. Don't try to make your life any better.

6. You know who is going to put you down for trying this and what they're going to say about you, so don't even bother.

Now that you've identified which one applies to you, you'll have to go back to the last chapter and do the accusation exercise for whichever one or ones apply to you with regard to how you deal with your frustrated needs.

Let Your Potential Live

Part 1: Expand Your Life Skills
Just by Making a Decision

Our goal today is to stimulate you to think about your challenges and your potential. Again, all you need to do is think about it, and to entertain the notion that you are wrong when you believe you can't do anything more to become the person you want to be. Making good changes in yourself and improving your life situation is part of an ever-evolving life flow. Getting back into this stream is what will help you conquer your emotional hunger. First let's do a broad survey of the ways you know you would like to improve your life. You're probably well aware of the big challenges looming in your life.

EXERCISE

Let Your Potential Live

Identify what parts of you are begging to be reborn by completing the sentence:

"It would make me feel better about myself if I _____."

use my business or career-related talents

use my creative talents

maintain commitments

become more romantic or sexual

use my leadership talents

become more loving and nurturing

become more religious or spiritual

become fun-loving and enjoy life

become independent

receive love and warmth

settle down

cooperate and be sensitive to others

become more moral

use my teaching talents

use my thinking abilities

Any area of personal development you chose from the list above is something you can do without anybody else's help or permission. All it takes is a decision to do it. All that is stopping you is your fear of failure. Think about any mistakes you've made or humiliations you've experienced. How did you feel when you failed or made a mistake in public? In private? Don't forget the small mistakes or embarrassments, such as asking "a stupid question" or coming in last in a race.

What was the end result of your mistake or failure? For instance, if you once had a terrible singing performance, did you stop singing? Or did you take lessons and improve? What does the way you handled your failure tell you? Have you avoided putting yourself forward in order to avoid the possibility of looking stupid again in public? What's the worst that might happen if you did look stupid? What do you fear? What opportunities have you missed by holding yourself back? How do you feel immediately after holding yourself back? What are the long-term effects?

If you actually spend a few moments thinking about these questions and possibly writing down your thoughts, you will discover a very bad cold feeling in the pit of your stomach. Note it well. It's not pleasant, but it is bearable. It's your shame/fear condensed into a small compact space felt somewhere inside what seems like your gut. It's easily converted into phantom hunger. If you could separate out the two feelings and become expert at distinguishing fear/shame from hunger, you would make another big step up in your conscious awareness and deal another big blow to your emotional eating habit. Once you can do this, you might be ready to reclaim some of your dreams that you've put in cold storage.

Part 2: Reclaim Your Personal Dreams

Remember what I said about passion and pleasure. If you don't find things to be passionate about in life, that creative energy that dwells in all of us will be forced into unproductive things like eating, arguing with your spouse, watching television constantly, and so on. Your life actually depends on you finding things that make your heart sing. Everyone has lists of things that they once dreamed about, everything from being president of the United States to flying to the moon to being a rock star. Some of those dreams may no longer be realistic but let's revisit those dreams for the sole purpose of using them to create new life goal dreams.

1. Think of two dreams you had when you were a child. For instance, maybe you wanted to be a teacher or an astronaut. Maybe you wanted to live in a castle and marry a prince or princess. Then list two dreams you had in your late teens or early twenties. Finally, list two dreams you have now. Don't worry about how far-fetched your dreams are. We will deal with that later.

2. Now write a list of things you love to do (everything from flipping the pages of a shiny magazine to singing), the things that you envy other people for doing. No one is going to see this list, so dream big.

3. Now look at your dreams. Consider them one by one, starting with your childhood dreams. If your dreams were not at all realistic, try to capture the grain of reality within them. For instance,

if you wanted to live in a castle when you were a kid, the adult version of that wish might translate to wanting to live in a beautiful home. If you wanted to be in a magical land, that might translate to having a mystical practice now and being surrounded by people who have similar interests. The dreams that honestly no longer interest you, cross off and accept that you are letting that one go.

4. Pick two dreams that you can actually begin to work toward achieving. For each one, break it into three parts, something you will do this week that will bring you closer to your dream, something you will do in six months, and then something you will do a year from now.

5. When you apply the Harriet Checklist, use the specific act you plan to do this week to get started on this dream.

EXERCISE

Harriet Checklist

Living your true potential, either your personal development issue from the list beginning on page 222 or the life goal dream you are considering, is one where Harriet has a field day. She loves to tell you how you can't try the things you secretly long to try. You can't dream. You can't hope. She is the ultimate party pooper, the rain on your parade, a real cynic. She basically tells you you're damned if you do and damned if you don't. If you try something and fail, you won't be able to live with yourself, and if you try something and succeed you'll be so full of yourself and people will be so envious that they'll leave you. You may not hear Harriet talking to you, saying these things, but you can be sure that she is down there stoking the fire on your fear and fueling your procrastination. If you believe all the things above that she has to say about you going after your dreams and goals, then you really only have the choice to eat. It is the only source of fulfillment you can expect. But if you see that all of this is just a projected fear, not a real fear, even though it feels real in the moment, you may be willing to try something anyway. After all, "courage is not the absence of fear, it's action in the face of fear." Think of a time when you felt something on you and thought it was a bug. In your belly you feel real fear, and then upon closer inspection you see that it is a leaf or a piece of lint and suddenly you feel better. The fears you have may feel really bad, but you can make yourself bigger than them if you find answers to Harriet's incessant chatter.

Let's pinpoint how Harriet has been playing a role in preventing you from living your true potential. Then go back to the accusation exercises in chapter 4 and start talking back. Anytime you are convinced that you shouldn't even bother giving your dreams a shot, Harriet has something to say about it.

You say: "In order to feel like I'm on my way to living my dreams, I am going to take an acting class." When you propose that, Harriet says to you one of the things from the list below.

1. You won't be able to do this perfectly, so you'd better not do it at all. If you do it, you will fail.

2. You have real faults, and everyone will know them if you try to do this. No one will want to be around you or with you.

3. You'll lose your protective armor and be out of control. Anything might happen. (Example: If I stop being a people-pleaser and focus on myself, people won't want to be around me.)

4. You have no right to aspire to anything more than you already have or to speak up for yourself.

5. You'd better not think your accomplishments or the compliments you get prove you're a good person. Don't try to make your life any better.

6. You know who is going to put you down for trying this and what they're going to say about you, so don't even bother.

Now that you've identified which one applies to you, you'll have to go back to the last chapter and do the accusation exercise for whichever one or ones apply to you with regard to how you deal with your unlived potential.

Be in Control of Your Stress, Don't Suffer from It

Stress is the enemy of all emotional eaters. Stress, broadly defined, involves everything we discuss in this book, so for our purposes I would like to focus on what you can do about it. First of all, be aware that you are already doing something about it as you explore the alternatives to powerlessness. Stress usually means we are temporarily overwhelmed with either too much to do or too many problems at the same time, leading to the feelings that trigger your eating pattern (see chapter 11, Session 2). It's the catastrophe predictions that create the overwhelmed experience. To the degree you have pinpointed them and started to master them, you have already cut down your stress load and your tendency to draw the powerlessness conclusion. When you go back to look at your notebook entries for Session 2, you'll find your list of stressors to use for this next exercise.

Personal Development and New Skills Are Key to Mastering Your Stress

Stress is caused by unsolved problems in living. You can better manage or resolve any problem in living if you are good at managing your money, your time, and your self-discipline. The exercise below will help you to identify ways to reduce your stress level by improving your day-to-day life skills.

EXERCISE

Mastering Your Stress

Select three items from the list below. Put them into categories (for example, money management, taking care of one's self, time management).

"To improve my day-to-day life I should _____."

make a budget

balance my checkbook

control spending and stay within my budget

pay bills and meet other financial commitments on time

make wise investments

plan for my retirement

plan for and pay my taxes

prioritize needs and desires and make purchases based on my priorities

define what it is I really want and need

let go of the security of being taken care of and stand on my own two feet

get the household chores done on a more regular basis

make plans and follow through on them

follow instructions or directions

discipline myself to complete my tasks

assemble appropriate tools and resources

frame and structure my day

establish and follow a schedule

set realistic deadlines or specific time limits

be on time for appointments and other commitments

accept help or support from others

frame and structure my day

allow myself the freedom not to be serious or responsible all the time

set goals that are within my reach

take care of my responsibilities so I can feel okay about having fun

schedule time for leisure activities or enjoyable events

schedule time to do what I want to do and feel entitled to establish realistic demands for myself

set more realistic deadlines or specific time limits

1. In your notebook, record the three improvements you need to make.

2. Under each improvement, write three to five bullet points describing how you will make that improvement, and by when.

3. Choose one bullet point to complete by tomorrow.

EXERCISE

Harriet Checklist

Dealing with stress is something that everyone must deal with. It's such a common issue because we as human beings get easily overwhelmed as we juggle so much and live in such uncertain times.

Let's pinpoint how Harriet has been playing a role in preventing you from powerfully dealing with stress. Remember that anything you chose on the list above is a life skill that will increase your autonomy, independence, and sense of adultness, as well as improve your self-esteem. And you know that your nagging critical conscience sees that as a threat. Anytime you back away from your personal development, you can be sure that Harriet's talking to you.

You say: "In order to feel more empowered with my daily responsibilities I am going to make a schedule and stick to it." When you propose that, Harriet says to you one of the things from the list below.

1. You won't be able to do this perfectly, so you better not do it at all. If you do it, you will fail.

2. You have real faults, and everyone will know them if you try to do this. No one will want to be around you or with you.

3. You'll lose your protective armor and be out of control. Anything might happen. (Example: If I stop being a people-pleaser and focus on myself, people won't want to be around me.)

4. You have no right to aspire to anything more than you already have or to speak up for yourself.

5. You'd better not think your accomplishments or the compli-
    ments you get prove you're a good person. Don't try to make
    your life any better.

6. You know who is going to put you down for trying this and
    what they're going to say about you, so don't even bother.

Now that you've identified which one applies to you, you'll have to
go back to the last chapter and do the accusation exercise for
whichever one or ones apply to you with regard to how you deal
with stress.

Don't Be Overwhelmed

In this session you've laid out and looked at all the hard work of
having a fulfilling adult life and fulfilling adult relationships. It may
seem like too much when it's all written down in your notebook, but
take some comfort in two facts.

First, you don't have to do everything at once. In fact, this is just
a list of ongoing life projects that you can do at your own pace.
Second, it's what everybody has to do when they become an adult.
Your list is not much different from that of all the people you know.
This is what you need to do to manage your life. If you don't do it,
who else is going to do it for you? I remember that when I first
started my psychiatric practice, young adults asked me what they
should do. I said, "I'll tell you how to lead your life if you'll do what
I tell you to do." Nobody ever took me up on that proposition. You
may think you want someone to take over for you, but you really
wouldn't let them even if they would. If you don't take charge, you'll
be frustrated like everyone else in a similar position. Don't fool yourself into believing that you can't do anything about it, so you have to
reward yourself with food. You can do these things. You can resume
your adult development and your journey toward autonomy. Your
phantom hunger will go away. You won't have to reward yourself
with food, because the work you'll be doing in your life will be
reward enough. If you choose not to do the work, you'll be frustrated
and want to eat. Remember, you're only fooling yourself. You don't

have to eat because these problems are unsolvable. They are solvable and you have a choice.

Stop Reinforcing Your Powerlessness

With regard to your frustration and feelings of being able to get rewarded in life, making a powerless choice looks like this: Something happens. There's a situation where you feel things are not going your way. You feel faced with too many obstacles and frustrations. This makes you feel defeated. One of the following things is happening.

- There's something not happening, or not happening when you want it to.
- There are obstacles making goals look too difficult to achieve.
- You have relationships that aren't going the way you want them to.
- You have needs that are not satisfied.
- You're aware of your unexplored potential and missed opportunities.
- You have too many stressors all at the same time.
- You've collected a series of failed attempts.

When any of those things happen you arrive at a misinterpretation: "I can't make my life work at all. I can't improve my relationships. I can't get my needs met. I can never reach my potential, and I can't develop the skills to master the stress in my life." Your frustrations make you feel powerless and you eat, seeking refuge in the food trance for a few moments. Then you feel guilty. Solving the problem with food confirms the fact that you can't make your life work. Let's see what this looks like in practice.

Powerless Choice Example

Liz tries out for the church choir and is not accepted (what happened in the external reality of today). She misinterprets what happens to believe that she can never get the things she wants and then it turns into a catastrophe prediction: she can't really sing at all (this happens in her internal reality, where things are weighed against her fears and past experiences). She goes immediately from the audition to a fast food restaurant, and when she's done she feels even more frustrated. Eating reinforces both her frustrations and her experience of powerlessness.

Powerful Reinterpretation   When something happens and you feel defeated, you have two choices: First, you can always recognize that you can try again. The second is that you can evaluate the situation based on what's happening today. You can see how else you can interpret what happened.

You can look for alternatives or adjust expectations.

You can accept that while obstacles are real, they can be worked with.

You can understand that relationships ebb and flow, and just because something is not going well doesn't mean it'll always be that way.

Getting needs satisfied happens between two people, and you have to figure out your part in it.

If a potential is not being fulfilled, perhaps it's not the right time or you need more training.

Handling stressors one at a time is less overwhelming.

A history of failures may be only a call for a fresh approach.

Powerful Reinterpretation Example   Liz tries out for the church choir and is not accepted. She thinks about what's really going on. She realizes that perhaps this wasn't the best time for her to be in the church choir, especially since her daughter is a senior in high school and will need a lot of her help this year. The choir is such a huge time commitment. Liz decides she'll use this year to take some voice lessons and will audition again next year. After thinking about things, Liz feels empowered and doesn't need to eat to deal with her frustration.

15

Creating Real Safety

In this session:

- You'll have to face the anxiety that you are hiding in the illusion of being safe or independent by being fat.
- You'll have to see how you eat more to feel safe but it doesn't make you safe, it just helps you avoid things and keeps you from recognizing the life decisions you've made that should be reviewed.
- You'll see that there are better ways to deal with the challenges you're hiding from other than using fat as a cover-up and excuse.
- You'll have to do the grown-up work in the real world that could actually get you real safety and real independence.
- You'll know that you have two methods besides arriving at the false conclusion that you're incapable of providing your own safety in life:
  1. You can use the insights you'll learn in this session to stop hiding so you can discover for yourself that you're not powerless.

2. You can stop misinterpreting the small dangers in your daily life that have added to your conclusion about powerlessness.

When we spoke about defeatism, you saw how your self-doubts and Harriet made you afraid to be the agent of your own life, made you afraid to try. You were so afraid and in need of a hiding place, and the hiding place you found was fat.

These exercises speak to the side of yourself that sabotages your efforts to diet, the part of you that wants you to stay fat, that actually uses your weight to prevent you from having the life you want. Most of this book has been dedicated to the rational side of yourself, the you that's fully committed to losing weight, that wants to have a healthy and attractive body, better relationships, and life fulfillment. But this other part of you, which I call the safety-seeking self, not only resists your efforts to diet, it's terrified of losing weight. It's almost as if you have two beings inside at odds with each other.

There is a part of you that feels powerless to create and maintain your own sense of safety without being overweight. You need to uncover how that part of you is thinking, and decide for yourself whether that makes any sense. I am convinced it doesn't, so let me show you why.

Identify What You're Trying to Hide under Your Fat

Look at the list below and see which ones you identify with.
"It serves me to stay fat _____."

because fat gives me an excuse to avoid contacts or make more overt efforts at meeting and being with people

so I can be more at ease with members of the opposite sex because there is no chance of a potential romance

because I don't have to deal with attention

because certain bodily or facial features will not be noticed if I am overweight

because I'll fail, and therefore I'd be worse off for trying (for example, going for a promotion, playing a sport, dancing, being an active parent)

because it is a way for me to have lower expectations of myself. (All of the items that you listed in chapter 5 are the things you have been avoiding as a way for you to decrease the demands you make on yourself.)

I'm sensitive to abandonment and rejection based on self-doubt and unloveability. (You've already dealt with this in chapter 4.)

because it controls certain impulses that I don't know how to control otherwise (for example, rage, tears, sex)

because I don't have to deal with my sexuality

because I don't have to be ambitious and perhaps disappointed

because it gives me an excuse to not express my need for closeness

because it helps me control my competitiveness with family members, friends, and colleagues

because it is a way for me to deal with my anger toward others

Fat doesn't bring you any real safety. It only helps you avoid knowing more fully what you already know to some degree, and keeps you from being clear about the decisions you have already made, which means you can't question them with the most conscious and intelligent part of your mind, so you remain stuck at a lower level of decision making.

Using fat this way is also a way of fooling yourself. You are not admitting to yourself that you have made certain decisions about the way you are now conducting your life.

Look at the items you chose from the list above. Now ask yourself whether being fat actually protects you from anything real. Are you not just fooling yourself about some fear-based decisions you have already made and are afraid to fully acknowledge? Wouldn't you be better off dealing with, rather than avoiding, the work needed to master

- shyness and fear of intimacy
- life challenges and opportunities
- self-doubts
- control of your impulses and passions

In this book, and in these sessions, I have already guided you to understand you are not powerless in these areas, so there is really no good reason to keep on avoiding facing them squarely and continuing your personal development. Here are some examples of the decisions you've already made and might want to rethink how you deal with.

- If you're using fat to avoid being sexually involved, then you've made a decision not to be sexually involved. Why not just accept that as fact and either stick to your decision (it's your right and your body), or reevaluate your decision and work on your fears? Either decision would be more clearly adult, and would make you a more powerful person. But using fat to avoid sexuality makes the whole decision process muddy.

- If you don't want sexual attention, just say no, or dress conservatively, or stay away from bars and clubs, or send out signals to your boss that you're unavailable.

- If you're shy, either work on it or accept it. Plenty of shy people do that without having to be overweight. Being overweight actually calls attention to yourself, which is the opposite of what most shy people consciously want.

- If you don't want to have affairs or be promiscuous, either decide to remain monogamous and stick to your decision, or figure out why you're looking outside your relationship, or why it feels impossible to remain committed.

- If it's intimacy, success, failure, or competition you fear, deal with it or live with it. There's no need to add fat to the equation. These are separate life course decisions that you have to

make or have already made that end up getting more complicated when you add fat to the mix. They need to be separated
out and dealt with for what they are, not covered over and
buried by food and fat cells.

It's better to own up to the decision and not be fat. Then you have
only that one problem to resolve: fat doesn't protect. It only covers
over a decision already made, and prevents an honest review of that
decision. It keeps you stuck. And being stuck means you're at least
temporarily powerless.

Here's where you are now. Here's how you've been keeping
yourself from a full awareness of the work you can and need to do.
Select the one that applies to you:

Overeating and being fat doesn't protect me from knowing
things, but it does prevent me from focusing on certain things
I can't or don't want to face.

Yes, being fat keeps me focused on the struggle to lose weight,
the guilt I feel when I fail, and how unattractive I am. Being
focused on those things protects me from feeling what I'm
really upset about.

Being engaged in the vicious cycle of overeating keeps things on
a surface level where I don't have to face the pain of the big
real issues. I know how to deal with my guilt and shame about
overeating—those are common feelings that every fat person
feels—but the other things make me feel too isolated, too
marginalized.

Do you want to stay in this state of avoidance knowing that it is
just avoidance, not real protection? You know that fat doesn't protect
you against impulse control, it simply provides you with a less
stigmatized impulse to control. For example, you may have been
shamed for your sexual impulses, and being fat may prevent you
from having to deal with sexual attention. While it may feel better to
be dealing with your impulse to overeat, just like so many other
people are, your need to be sexually self-expressed doesn't really go
away by staying fat, it just gives you another frustrated need.

Maintain Your Old Role in the Family or Emerge as Yourself

As I described in chapter 6, the safety chapter, there is a deeper layer of fear related to your family of origin. Whenever you take up a life challenge and personal development task rather than avoiding it, you're unconsciously changing your role relationship to your family of origin because you're actively charting your own path through life, realizing your own potential, and becoming who you really are, rather than who you used to be. If you stay stuck in the roles you've been assigned or assigned yourself, you'll feel frustrated, but you'll also feel safe. Every role we occupy is connected to people, both past and present, and all these people have a stake in you remaining in your familiar role. Stepping out of your role is necessary but dangerous, both real danger that comes from disrupting social patterns, but mostly exaggerated danger that accompanies the individuation quest.

EXERCISE

Identify Your Role in Your Family

Look at the list below and think about which roles were assigned to you or accepted by you in your family and which ones were given to your siblings.

athlete	alcoholic
brain	bad-tempered one
drama queen	oversexed one
most likely to succeed	bad student
beauty	shy one
hunk	stubborn one
black sheep	ugly one
angry one	caretaker
rejected and unloved one	troublemaker
favored	peacemaker

Judi was a typical late 1950s teenager. She wore poodle skirts and cardigans. She dated nice boys and was a good student. Her sister Marlee would never get noticed in the family if she were so similar to Judi. So Marlee became the black sheep. She dyed her blond hair black and dated college guys with motorcycles. She's now in her sixties, but she still maintains the family role of the rebel.

You and everyone you know fit some role stereotype like these while growing up. These assigned roles are our family legacy and control much of what we do and how we think about ourselves until the time that we emerge from them. Most of us do emerge completely over time, but some don't. When fat is used as a hiding place, the emergence is prolonged.

Family-assigned roles distort who you are and limit who you're capable of being. That's why there is such a strong drive to transcend these roles. They're not sacred and fixed. They can be questioned, altered, or given up. But you have to fight hard to do this and ultimately become the one in charge of who you are and how your life works.

The real danger of stepping out of a family role and reclaiming yourself is the danger of being punished, ostracized, and envied by others. You fear being talked about, labeled, and excommunicated from the clan. When you lose weight and become intent on remaking your life, you expose yourself to these ancient anxieties. Your critical conscience tells you that you can feel safe again only if you get fat again.

EXERCISE

Remodeling Your Family Role

Look at the most important family-assigned role you've been working on changing (everyone is always working on at least one). Ask yourself these questions:

> If I make the changes I want to make, would I really face unbearable punishment or be ostracized immediately and irrevocably, either by family, friends, or co-workers?

If there were some real threat or real danger incurred by doing this, could I work it out if I approached it with an open mind and mature adult perspective?

Can I separate the real consequences from my catastrophic predictions that have been keeping me from fully emerging?

If, in the previous exercises, you've come to the conclusion that fat doesn't make you safe, then of course it's not worth paying the price for an empty illusion of feeling safe. But in case you still think fat gives you some real protection other than just avoidance, think about whether the protection you get is worth the price of being fat. Make a list of what fat costs you in your life. We can start you out with the obvious:

"Using fat as a source of safety means I won't be able to

_____."

feel like an adult who can make empowered choices

solve problems

feel loveable

feel worthy

be healthy

earn the respect and admiration of others

live a fulfilled life

be seen for who I really am

Being overweight has surely protected you from some very frightening emotions and core beliefs, but it has cost you a lot. One way to retreat from center stage, to allay expectations, is to get fat. As we mentioned on page 98, people suffer from being fat. They suffer salary discrimination, they are not considered for promotions, and they are exempt entirely from certain areas of employment. Fat people also suffer in the area of relationships. Taking all of these things into consideration, you might want to ask yourself if being fat is really worth the illusion of safety that it provides.

Real Ways to Feel Safe

If you apply only a half-mindful effort to your career or marriage because you want to avoid certain pieces of psychological work or difficult decisions, if you hide behind fat in these arenas in order to "duck out," your marriage and your work will be less likely to continue successfully in a way that's satisfying.

You can increase your real safety in the world by facing reality, looking for real dangers, anticipating problems, and looking for solutions. You can keep your relationships strong and invest yourself in good people who are trustworthy, decent, and well put together. You can avoid impulsive big decisions like falling in love and marrying before you really know the real person, or marrying the wrong person to spite your parents. There are hundreds of things you can do and skills you can further develop to provide yourself as much safety as possible in what is at times an unpredictable world. But to be your own adult provider of real safety, you have to face reality, whatever it is, and work with it. When you hide in fat to give yourself the illusion of safety by avoiding challenge, you're not facing up to reality, and you are missing the opportunity to take charge of your own safety and make it as real as possible.

Create Real Safety

Now make your own list of what you can do to give yourself real safety in the world, using the principles I outlined above. First, look at the areas in your life where you feel vulnerable, for example, a relationship, your finances, your health or someone else's health, or your children. Now address each of those with what you know could and should be done to make you be more safe, not just feel safe. For example: You see that the family finances are very uncertain, you're concerned that you won't have enough money for your child's college fund, and you know that you can and you should go back to work to begin earning that money. Up until now, you've just been worrying about it and hoping that your spouse could make you feel safe with the statement, "Everything will work out somehow." You finally see that only taking an action that changes the situation can provide real safety.

Stop Reinforcing Your Powerlessness

With regard to your feeling safe in life, making a powerless choice looks like this: Something happens. There's a situation where you feel like you're stepping out of a familiar role. This makes you feel scared, and you look for a place to hide. One of the following things may be happening.

> You have an opportunity to perform at a higher level, either at work or at play.
>
> You're in the spotlight for some reason.
>
> Your passions are aroused and you're tempted to act on them.
>
> You're making a life course decision.
>
> You're beginning to admire and enjoy people not usually accepted by your family or spouse.
>
> You're caught up in a past experience where you were abused or hurt, or something similar to what happened in the past is happening now.

When any of those things happen you're likely to arrive at a misinterpretation: "I can't protect myself. I expect to be punished for daring to change. I expect to be attacked, falsely labeled, humiliated, embarrassed, put down, or expelled from the family." Your fears make you feel powerless and you eat, seeking refuge in the food trance for a few moments, and then you feel guilty. Using food in this way confirms the fact that you can't possibly deal with life in a brave way. Let's see what this looks like in practice.

Powerless Choice Example

Marissa is in an unsatisfying and almost verbally abusive relationship (what's happening in her external reality of today). She misinterprets her relationship to believe she's better off with him than alone. She fears that her family would never approve of her decision to leave him; after all, her family role is the martyr. She fears she won't be able to manage money on her own, and then it turns into a catastrophe prediction: I was abused as a child and this relationship is not nearly as bad. Perhaps this is the best treatment I can expect from those who love me (this happens in her internal reality, where things are weighed against her fears and past experiences). Marissa can't find the courage to leave her husband, but she's created a separation from him by gaining two hundred pounds. Being fat reinforces both her lack of safety and her experience of powerlessness.

Powerful Reinterpretation   There are two ways to transform your experience of powerlessness. You can dialogue with Harriet, who tells you that you must hide yourself and avoid being the agent of your life because you're not really an adult (accusation #4), or you can reassess the situation rather than make an immediate misinterpretation that reinforces your powerlessness. Marissa needs to analyze the situation based on what's happening today. You can assess a situation where you're afraid and don't know how to create a sense of safety in one of the following ways:

You can assess the real risk and reward of your decision.

You can value your own opinion over the opinions of others.

You can deflect others' feelings of envy by understanding that it's a form of flattery.

You can work toward creating real safety.

You can bravely adopt a new role that's different from your family role of the past.

You can learn to maintain boundaries.

Powerful Reinterpretation Example   Marissa is in an unsatisfying and almost verbally abusive relationship. She thinks about what's really going on. She realizes that she's done all the work she can possibly do, she's asked her husband to go to couples counseling, she's altered her own attitude (she did this in the frustration/reward layer), and her husband is unwilling to make any compromises. She realizes that while getting divorced and living on her own will be difficult, she can't continue to hide under layers and layers of fat. She realizes that only by having her own home will she be safe from his constant barrage of abusive comments. After thinking about things, Marissa feels empowered by deciding to move out, and she no longer needs her fat to hide beneath.

16

SESSION 7
Maturely Dealing
with Anger

In this session:

- You'll identify how you deal with your own anger, so you don't have to eat to control it.

- You'll see how by eating to deal with anger, you're attacking yourself rather than anyone else.

- You'll recognize that eating to defy or punish someone only gives you the false feeling of power, and that's not real independence.

- You'll learn the six different ways that you mask or excuse using food and fat as an aggressive weapon.

- You'll see that you can recover your power by becoming more skilled at expressing anger appropriately in the context of very specific situations. You'll identify who you have grievances with.

- You'll have to remember that you have two methods to void your powerless conclusion about anger and eating:

1. Remember that rebellion and defiance are not the same as healthy independence and autonomy.
2. Stop adding to your anger by confusing old anger with current situations.

The next tricky reason you overeat is to rebel. Often you might be getting back at a parent, a partner, or someone else in your past. Sometimes you're taking things out on your own body because it feels safer than showing your anger and defiant attitude, and risking abandonment. Sometimes it's just your way of throwing up your hands when frustrated and expressing your anger through a kind of primitive defiance: "If I can't control my world, I can at least hurt myself." You, like most people, find it difficult to give up your blame in order to accept full responsibility for overcoming the past, exercising your resilience, and making your life work despite past battles. Letting go of revenge and anger is hard, but it's what you must do if you ever want to truly grow up. Eating to rebel is a drama played out upon yourself, only incidentally and peripherally exacting revenge on others. Let's look at how this drama plays out in the familiar forms of eating rebellion. We talked about them in depth in part one; now let's look at what you can do about them.

1. Love me first, and then I will lose weight.
2. They made me this way, so I can't change.
3. I'll get back at them.
4. I am not this body.
5. Food is my only pleasure, so I'm not going to give it up.
6. I can't be perfect, so I'd rather be fat.

Love Me First, and Then I Will Lose Weight

When one feels unworthy of love, they put their partner through many tests in an effort to get their partner to prove how much they are loved. Being fat may seem to be a good test. Your spouse should, after all, love you just the way you are, right? But you may want to ask yourself who your weight is really punishing.

Are you treating your current or former romantic partner in this unrealistic way—asking them to love the fat that you hate? Asking them to be the unconditional loving object? When you expect or demand that they treat you with unconditional love, you're asking the impossible in order to replay an image you have about "others" who say they love you, and this image was generated in the home you grew up in. You partner will always lose. If he or she seems to love you when you're fat and you decide to lose weight, he or she might like it. Then you pounce on that and say they like you more thin than fat, therefore they were lying to you when you were fat, so you get fat again to punish the hypocrite and deceiver. This will always keep you fat and your partner off-balance. You'll always be angry and mistrustful. What you need to keep in mind is that this is not about you and him, it is about the way you felt a long time ago and the parent who you think didn't love you in the right way.

EXERCISE

Is It Your Partner or Your Parent?

What you need to do to stop this pattern is use the insight above and write out the conversation you would like to have had with that parent who didn't give you the unconditional love you wanted (you don't actually have to give what you wrote to the parent who disappointed you). You should do this to keep the past separate from the current conversation you need to have with your partner. With your partner, you need to explain the pattern you've been producing, ask him or her to be understanding about why you've done this in the past, and make a commitment to him or her to not do it again in the future. That'll help you sort out the real world from the old tapes that keep you defying your own best judgment about food in order to play out this angry, mistrustful scenario. Tell him about how you feel with regard to being overweight, and how you wouldn't expect him to say it's all right when it's not, and that you know real love is based on honest feedback and honest self-awareness.

They Made Me This Way,
So I Can't Change

Perhaps you've stayed overweight because "your parents made you this way" by overfeeding you or using food alternatively as a reward or a punishment. Perhaps you even say that there's a genetic component to your weight, so that they literally "made you this way." If you're still using your weight to get back at your parents, you're giving them far too much power over your life. Remember, they don't rule you anymore, you do. It's your anger that's keeping them in power in your head. You don't give up your blame and anger, but you don't express it directly, either, so you act it out on yourself through overeating, having a fictional argument with parents who are not there to listen or answer back, and are not there to be hurt. When you keep this pattern up, it means you're scared of your anger and don't know what to do with it other than hurt yourself and give yourself some illusion that you're punishing them through your suffering. Although it may be true that that works on some parents, I have seen people perpetuate this pattern long after their parents were dead.

EXERCISE

Why Are Your Parents Still in Charge?

You need to recognize that this is an internal drama and work on stepping outside this drama into the real world. Who did this to you, and what did they really do? Even if you were too young to reject this parenting and feeding, what makes you still think that you have to accept this historical fact as the final statement about you and your body? Use your Harriet Dialogues to talk to the ghosts within you. Give yourself back the ultimate authority over your life. Recognize that you're keeping this up with your unexpressed anger and blame, and that only you are being hurt. If you have real grievances with your parents, then either decide to air them out, or let go of them. Either way is better than eating yourself into poor health.

I'll Get Back at Them

This one builds on the last one. Not only does it make your parents responsible for the way you are today, but it adds a component of punishment for their parental failures. You have dedicated your life and are using your body to frustrating them at any cost.

EXERCISE

Do You Want to Use Your Body as a Battlefield?

Do you still harbor anger at parents who didn't treat you well as a child? Are they still doing it? If so, do you want to tell them how angry you are? Are you afraid to do it or not sure it's right or wise? In any case, looking at and deciding what you want to do in the circumstances of now is much better (even if you do nothing) than continuing holding a grudge and acting out on yourself a silent revenge (even if it annoys them to this day). Look at the difference between now and then. Don't be afraid to feel your hurt and anger and then decide what to do with it. If you don't, your anger will eat you up, a totally futile, harmful, and useless thing to do with your life. Just recognize that you have been using your body as a weapon of revenge, and ask yourself if that is what you still want to do.

I Am Not This Body

Perhaps for you, due to a history of physical or sexual abuse, you decided that being in your body was not a safe place to be. You may have separated from your body as a way to protect yourself, but time has passed and you're safe now. When it happened, you were over-whelmed and flooded with feelings, fears, and guilt. Now you can sort this out. You can protect yourself from more abuse. You can deal with the emotions that come up through insight and understanding, and counseling if necessary. You have to find ways to begin to invite yourself back in. If, however, you are in a situation where you are still being abused, please get help.

Reclaiming Your Body

While it may not have felt like your body for a long time, it *is* your body. Try these three techniques for increasing body awareness when something upsets you:

1. Spend 5 minutes at a time looking in a full-length mirror, talking to yourself.

2. Slow down your breathing. Remember to breathe from your diaphragm. Make sure that you take complete breaths. Focus all your attention on your breath.

3. Get into a bathtub and massage yourself. Better yet, get someone else to massage you. Pay attention to each part of your body as it gets touched.

These are the physical acts you can do to start the reunion process, but remember, it is a psychological journey that has to happen, and it's a return to the natural state of being, so your own body will get you there if you give it a chance. Fat only separates you from yourself, and defying yourself in order to stay fat is just another way of expressing your anger at what happened and maintaining the split that makes you feel safe, as if you were not now older and more capable of handling the emotions of the past.

Food Is My Only Pleasure, So I'm Not Going to Give It Up

In chapter 14 (Session 5), you got to see how food can never fill the place of real pleasure. It cannot love you, it cannot make you proud, it cannot get you the affection, attention, and acknowledgment that you so deeply crave. That's a fact. There is another fact: when you say to yourself that food is your only or last pleasure, you're operating off an image of yourself that you should question. Are you really so ruined as a person that you can't get pleasure from relationships and the abundant opportunities in life? Is it true that only an inanimate thing, food, is capable of satisfying you, filling you up? Do you recognize that this is the angriest statement of all regarding food, that it says the whole world is useless to you? No one can provide you with the pleasure that food does?

EXERCISE

Finding Real Pleasure

What you need to do now is prove to yourself that this image of yourself—as a person who can get fulfillment only out of food—is an old image you fell into and perpetuated out of habit by not looking closely at yourself. It's not who you really are. It is an idea about yourself that has grown out of your disappointment. Perhaps in earlier chapters you began to outline what you really have been craving in your life. Take three things and begin making them a reality this week. Pay special attention to the pleasure you get from doing the things you've put off doing.

I Can't Be Perfect, So I'd Rather Be Fat

Once again, I'd like to remind you that you'll never be perfect—no one will. It's a hard ideal to give up, but it's one that every happy, successful person must at some point let go of. Be aware that this is a colossal excuse, and the aggression is directly toward your own critical conscience, Harriet. You're eating to defy her because she has you believing you must be perfect in order to accept yourself and be acceptable to others. If you're still addicted to being perfect, please revisit the Harriet dialogues in chapter 13 (Session 4).

EXERCISE

Putting Perfection in Perspective

Dialogue with Accusation #1 in Session 4, chapter 13.

EXERCISE

Mature Ways to Handle Anger

You'll have to rely on the principle that we've repeated many times in this book: Look to the reality of the situation, and start by assuming that all realities are complex and open to multiple interpretations. You have to be a "reality detective" and analyze each clue, and only after that decide on a response. You'll have to accept that your first blush of anger is a reflex based on a misinterpretation that the old anger situation and the current anger situation are the same. That needs to be followed by a thinking pause so you can see the difference. In that pause you can choose a mature way to deal with your anger. Choose a new way to handle a specific anger situation maturely.

You can use it to motivate yourself.

You can clear up a misunderstanding.

You can admit your responsibility in the matter.

You can compromise.

You can interpret envy as flattery.

You can discover that the act against you was unintentional.

You can realize that your sense of entitlement or expectations is what led you to feeling angry.

You can assert in an appropriate way your rights and reasonable expectations.

True independence comes from acting appropriately, wisely, and maturely according to your own values of what is right and wrong. The more you keep your anger response keyed to the specifics of a particular reality situation, the more powerful you will be as a person. That will eliminate your defiant eating patterns.

EXERCISE
Address Grievances or Give Them Up

Everyone has a list of people who have hurt or disappointed them throughout their life, beginning with their ancestors who determined their physical features and genetics, to their parents, to the person who just cut them off driving 5 minutes ago. In your notebook, make a list of people you have grievances against. Like I helped you to do with your unmet needs, we need to find a resting place for these grievances so that you can address them in an empowered way or let them go.

1. Have a conversation with or go to counseling with the person.
2. Own your responsibility in the grievance.
3. Make a decision that resolution cannot be made with this particular person (either because they're dead, they're not in your life anymore, or they're unwilling), and let it go.

Stop Reinforcing Your Powerlessness

With regard to your ability to deal with anger in life and how that makes you rebel, making a powerless choice looks like this: Something happens. There's a situation that makes you feel angry and vengeful. One of the following things may have happened:

You've been disrespected.

You don't feel appreciated.

You feel misunderstood.

You feel used.

You feel abused.

You feel belittled.

You feel betrayed.

When any of those things happen you're likely to arrive at a misinterpretation: "I don't know how to handle my anger." Suppressing your anger makes you feel powerless, and you eat because by chewing on food you avoid a confrontation and the possibility of "biting someone." Let's see what this looks like in practice.

Powerless Choice Example

John, as a child, always felt like his mother was more interested in other things besides him: her magazines, her needlepoint, talking on the phone, going shopping, soap operas, you name it. Feeding him was the only way she offered him any kind of attention. She made his favorite meals and sat down at the table to eat with him. John has been overweight his whole life. He recently went on JDate, an online dating service. He put a photo up from when he weighed less. He had been having a nice correspondence with Ruth for about three weeks, but when he finally met her, she seemed disappointed, and came right out and said he was too fat (what happened in the external reality of today). John is angry and misinterprets what Ruth said to believe that he'll never get a date. He calls his mother and says it's her fault that he's fat, and then it turns into a catastrophe prediction: I'll never find a woman who'll love me. (This happens in his internal reality, where things are weighed against his fears and past experiences.) John ends up eating to get back at Ruth, and at his mother for making him fat in the first place. How eating can possibly punish either one of them is illogical from the outside, but makes sense at the time he's doing it. Being fat reinforces both his rebelliousness and his experience of powerlessness.

Powerful Reinterpretation   There are two ways to transform your experience of powerlessness. You can dialogue with Harriet, who migrates into other people to confirm your own self-doubts (accusation #6), or you can reassess the situation rather than make an immediate misinterpretation that reinforces your powerlessness. John needs to analyze the situation based on what's happening today. You can assess a situation where you're angry and think of other ways to deal with that anger rather than rebelling. You can handle it in one of the following ways:

Communicate and clear up any misunderstandings.

Learn breathing techniques.

Own your responsibility for how things went wrong.

Make amends with people from the past so you're not harboring the resentment of old grievances.

Forgive when you can.

Powerful Reinterpretation Example   John recently went on JDate, an online dating service. He put a photo up from when he weighed less. He had been having a nice correspondence with Ruth for about three weeks but when he finally met her, she seemed disappointed, and came right out and said he was too fat. He thinks about what's really going on. John realizes that he was deceptive to put up that photo in the first place and that Ruth had a right to feel disappointed. He also realizes that while his mother didn't provide him with the attention he needed as a child, he's limiting the possibility of a real relationship with her today by harboring an old resentment. Finally, he realizes that by eating he's only hurting himself; he's not really getting back at anyone. After all, being so spiteful is not such an attractive quality. John sends Ruth an e-mail apologizing. She's so touched by his honesty that she agrees to stay in touch with him. They start biking together and John is finally losing weight effortlessly. They agree on things, they laugh, and he's finally getting the attention from a woman that he always longed for.

17

SESSION 8
Fill Yourself Up

In this session:

- You'll understand your experience of emptiness to see exactly what it means to you and how you can take charge of your life to deal with it so you don't have to keep trying to fill yourself up with food.

- You'll understand the mystery layer of emptiness. You'll identify your abandonment fear and see it for what it is, an outdated image and memory of what you feared as a child.

- You'll become intimately acquainted with your expectancy pattern and the catastrophe prediction you make about being deprived or disappointed.

- You'll have to prove to yourself, by the experience of catching yourself, that your expectancy pattern is not the right way to deal with your relationships in life.

- You'll have to stop adding to your emptiness by mistrusting what is being given to you by those who love you.

- You'll have to remember that you have two methods to void your powerlessness conclusion about emptiness:
  1. Remember that emptiness can never be filled with food.
  2. Stop adding to your feelings of emptiness by confusing your childhood fear of abandonment with current situations.

EXERCISE

What Does the Experience of Emptiness Mean to You?

For every person, emptiness is different. You'll need to determine when you specifically feel empty. "I feel empty when _____."

Self-Doubt Layer

I am filled with self-doubts

I don't feel good enough about myself

I feel judged

Frustration/Reward Layer

I feel unsatisfied in my relationships

I'm lonely

I'm far from people I love

my needs aren't met

I am not involved in something I'm passionate about

I'm overwhelmed and can't manage my life

Safety Layer

I'm anxious

I'm having conflict with my family

I'm scared to try something new

Rebellion Layer

I feel misunderstood

I feel alienated

I feel marginalized or unimportant

Emptiness Layer

I am in a moment where life doesn't make sense

I'm with people I love, but I don't feel like I fit in

I'm going through a big change in life

I feel as if I never get my expectations met by anyone

Look at which categories your feelings of emptiness fall into, and that's how you'll determine the work you need to do. If how you feel falls into one of the first four categories go back, and work in those areas. If how you feel falls into the last category (the emptiness layer), then proceed through this session and I'll show you how to work with those feelings.

Understanding the Fear of Abandonment

In chapter 8, you saw how the fear of abandonment is our most deeply ingrained and oldest fear and that it often leads to feelings of emptiness that you try to fill with food. You also saw how your child-hood fear of abandonment can exacerbate your current day fear of abandonment. It's normal for you to be afraid that the people you love—your parents, your partner, your friends, your children—will go away or die. But these fears become unbearable when they're associated with our old fears of abandonment. Let's separate those out now. In your notebook, draw two columns. On the top of the lefthand column, write "Old Abandonment Fears," and on the other one write "Current Abandonment Fears."

On your list of "Old Abandonment Fears," write out times when you feared you were abandoned, times when people stopped being your friend as a child, when someone died or moved away, or any nightmares or fears you had. Explore the feelings and what you did with them. On your list of "Current Abandonment Fears," write down your current fears such as someone getting sick or dying, relationships breaking up, an anticipated move, children moving away, and so forth.

EXERCISE

Abandonment Fears

Look at the lists side by side. Here's what you should ask yourself about your current abandonment fears: "How can I find a resting spot for these fears?"

You can find a resting spot by asking:

1. Can this abandonment be prevented? If so, how? (For instance, if someone has a life-threatening illness and they're not taking good care of themselves medically, they can get treatment.)

2. Can this abandonment be prepared for? If so, how? (For instance, if your children will be going away to college soon, you can begin to develop your own interests and activities so that when they're gone, your life is full.)

3. If a certain abandonment can't be prevented or prepared for, then how will you cope with it? For instance, if you're going through a divorce, you can make sure you have appropriate support systems and good legal counsel.

When you look at the two lists side by side, can you identify ways in which your old fears intensify your current abandonment fears? Simply identifying them will be enough to awaken a new awareness.

In chapter 8, you saw that you may still be longing for the people in your life to love you the way a parent loves an infant, immediately attending to their every need. However, back then your needs were simple. You needed to be picked up when you cried and fed when you were hungry. Even at that early time, you began to form images in your mind about what to expect when you were in need of human contact. Each mother–child relationship sets in motion an expectancy pattern for all relationships to come. If you recognize within you (this may not be true for everyone or to the same degree) a tendency to mistrust the love that's given to you, to hold yourself back in an effort to be self-protective, or to constantly be disappointed by the people who are meant to love you, then you may have an expectancy pattern that is creating your feelings of emptiness. If when you're being loved you don't accept it, then it doesn't fill you up.

EXERCISE
Observe

You'll need to find a way to put that expectancy pattern aside, acknowledge when you're getting real love, and let the warmth of real love fill you up without being afraid. The way you do that is to catch yourself in those moments when you know you're being loved but don't let it happen. For example, your spouse tries to make you feel good when you're in a bad mood, and instead of getting annoyed, as if to say that what he/she is doing isn't enough, you pause and tell your partner that you appreciate the effort that's being made.

EXERCISE
What Fills You Up?

You'll need to ask yourself what really fills you up. Look into your past and see which moments in your life felt full of meaning—moments when you felt awake, present, loved, seen, known. "I feel full when _____."

I'm in love

I get a good report at work

I feel like my life is on track

I feel connected to God

all my loved ones are happy and healthy

I'm passionately engaged in something

I'm connecting with someone

I'm taking care of myself

I'm taking care of others or engaged in some kind of service

Make your own list full of specific situations (the more specific you make them, the better), so that you can refer to it at times when you feel overwhelmed with a feeling of emptiness.

Stop Reinforcing Your Powerlessness

With regard to your feeling fulfilled in life, making a powerless choice looks like this: Something happens. There's a time or situation or person that leaves you feeling empty. The emptiness is so uncomfortable that you immediately seek to try to fill it with food. One of the following things may be happening:

Someone is holding a grudge against you.

A loved one has died.

A relationship has ended.

You don't feel loved by anyone.

You're not appreciated.

You're far away from those that you feel connected to.

Nothing in your life makes sense.

When any of those things happen, you may arrive at a misinterpretation: "I'll never feel loved or fulfilled. Nobody understands me. I'm all alone in the world." Your emptiness makes you feel powerless, and you eat to momentarily have a tangible feeling of fullness. Let's see what this looks like in practice.

Powerless Choice Example

Denise's boyfriend left her. They had been making plans to get married. While Denise was on a business trip in Denver, Alan packed up all his things and left. When she returned home, his closets were empty (what's happening in her external reality of today). She misinterprets this to mean she'll never be properly loved, and then it turns into a catastrophe prediction: My father died when I was ten, men always leave me, I'll always be alone (this happens in her internal reality, where things are weighed against her fears and past experiences). Denise starts eating all the time. She just can't stand that empty feeling in her gut. In six months, she's gained forty pounds. Eating reinforces her emptiness by intercepting her ability to look for things that would really fill her up and confirms her experience of powerlessness.

Powerful Reinterpretation   There are two ways to transform your experience of powerlessness. You can dialogue with Harriet, who tells you that you're not perfect, so you're not good (accusation #1), or you can reassess the situation rather than make an immediate misinterpretation that reinforces your powerlessness. Denise needs to analyze the situation based on what's happening today. You can assess a situation where you feel empty and don't know how to create a real sense of fullness in one of the following ways:

> You can ask for forgiveness.
>
> You can form new relationships.
>
> You can get grief counseling.
>
> You can accept that your abandonment fears of yesterday are different from your abandonment fears of today.
>
> You can stop expecting people to provide you with the unconditional love of a parent.
>
> You can find ways to connect with people or activities.

Powerful Reinterpretation Example   Denise's boyfriend left her. They had been making plans to get married. While Denise was on a business trip in Denver, Alan packed up all his things and left. When she returned home, his closets were empty. Alan was not even willing to discuss why he left. He just says that it's what he needs to do. Denise stops and thinks about what's really going on. She realizes that her feelings are made worse by the fact that her father died and "left" when she was ten. She dialogues with Harriet and accepts that just because Alan left doesn't mean that she is deeply flawed or that she'll always be alone. The pain of her emptiness forces her to get counseling, where she discusses not only the pain of losing her relationship but also the pain of her father's death. Only then does Denise realize how her father's death and her fear of abandonment have been affecting all her adult relationships. She had been holding back and not really loving her partners the way they were loving her. After all, she was too afraid because they might leave. When Denise begins to do this adult work to fill her emptiness, she feels empowered, she doesn't need to eat to make herself feel full, and she finally can see that the chance for a fulfilling relationship can be possible.

Shrink Yourself
Conclusion

By now you've done a lot of work. You've thought a lot. You've explored a lot. You may still feel overwhelmed and long for a simple magical solution to losing weight and having the body you want. We all long for an easy way out, and I wish I could've offered you that, but it simply wasn't an option. Taking your power back, one choice at a time, is in fact the only way to take control of your weight forever.

As you practice these skills in your life, you may at first be able to handle one of the five layers with ease while still having trouble with emptiness or some other layer. I explain to my patients that this doesn't mean they haven't progressed, it just means that there are areas where they've been more dependent on food. And those areas require more time, more patience, and more perseverance. You may at first be able to control your afternoon snacking at work, but not your nighttime bingeing. Whatever areas are still challenging for you are only indications of where you need to do deeper work—where you need to ask more questions, make more choices, reinterpret, dialogue with Harriet, or look more closely. Managing your life is a lifetime project, and mastering your relationship with food is just one very important project within that project.

Ultimately, your goal should be to catch yourself every time before you overeat, to find that pause between when something happens and when you have the uncontrollable urge to eat. In that pause is where the real you lives—the person who has dreams, feelings, ideas, needs, goals, and unfulfilled potential—the person who has been kept down all this time with food. When you don't eat, you allow that person, the real you inside, to emerge, and then your life can be full of possibility and you can finally have the body you want.

At www.shrinkyourself.com you'll find the Hunger Coach, a program that will help you capture that pause before you overeat.

There isn't much more to say except to remind you of the obvious (which I always find to be the most important):

- It's your life and only you can make it work.

- It's better to have the power of self-determination than to give away your power to your own primitive conscience. A mature conscience makes life a hell of a lot easier.

- As the adult author of your life, you can write the book any way you want.

Index